My Garden Journal

A monthly guide to healthier food

By Rita Engelken

My Garden Journal

Copyright © 1996 by Rita Engelken

Printed by G & R Publishing Company
507 Industrial Street
Waverly, Iowa 50677

All rights reserved. This book may not be reproduced in whole or in part in any form whatsoever without written permission except in the case of brief quotations embodied in critical articles and reviews.

Printing History
First G & R Publishing Company printing 1996

Printed in the United States of America.

INTRODUCTION

This is a book about growth. At the most obvious level, Rita Engelken is writing about the chores which each gardener faces with each passing month. But for Rita, gardening is never really separated from living or from believing. It is all one. She lives her life as she believes, and through the blend of faith and practice the world has paid her back. Now she is sharing it with you in these pages.

Towards the end of her book she makes note of how she has taught farmers in Canada, Lativia and Siberia on the value of composting. My personal involvement with Rita includes those experiences in Lativa and Siberia, when she was part of delegations of sustainable farmers who helped to develop the programs of my organization, REAP International. I can tell you that Rita did much more than teach farmers how to compost.

I have a vivid memory of Rita in Lativia. We held a conference which was attended by equal numbers of farmers and academics. The academics were primarily from the Latvian Agricultural Academy -- which is their version of an Iowa State or Cornell University. Rita's lecture was full of personal references to her family, to the problems they had with pesticides, to the changes in her life. There were facts too, but always from the heart. I watched the Latvians, who were just feeling the first breeze of freedom and optimism in their county, listening to this Iowa farm woman. It was difficult for me to tell how they would react. Then at the end of her talk, a spokesman rose to provide an evaluation of her talk. He was a professor from the academy. He summarized her lecture and thanked her for sharing her personnel experiences. His concluding remark said it all: "I have learned more from listening to Mrs. Engelken for a few hours," he said, "then I have from a semester in any one of our academic classes."

In the following pages, you will learn about compost. You will learn when to do things and what you should do. But you will also learn about a woman who has experienced a lifetime of growth through her garden, the people close to her, and the land on which she lives.

Rita's is a classic American story. She came from a humble family. She grew up during the Depression. Her large family had to scrape to make ends meet. It was a style of life which she took with her into marriage. She and her husband Ralph began their farming with the so-called conventional wisdom of the day. They used pesticides and synthetic fertilizers in the same ways as their neighbors. But the price they paid was the health of their children. The toxins in their environment brought sores to the children. At that time, they were fortunate to have the counsel of Father Louie White, who advised them on ways to farm which would improve their health and that of the land itself. Over the years, they heeded his advice. But it was not easy. They faced skepticism from other farmers and from academics, who could not believe that their system worked. That is why it was very interesting in Latvia to watch another group of academics and their reaction to her. She had come full circle, with a very different conclusion.

In the pages of her book, Rita maps out how she came to have her vision - - a way to look at the world. It is a modest vision, which does not draw attention to itself, but it is there nonetheless. Like the seasons itself, it comes in little things which she looks forward to and which are important to the cycle. To all things there is a season.

I know that Rita would tell you that by reading her book, you will learn how to garden. But you may also learn how to live. "I think of my life as a crusader to prove health can be restored to soil and in turn make the world healthier in which to live," she writes.

William Mueller
Director
Rural Enterprise Adaptation Program

August 28, 1996

FOREWORD

As I prepared these pages of my journal, memories were brought back to me when I was a child learning from my mother the skills of growing our own food. I was born in the years of the depression, so raising food was a necessity with most families then. We canned most of our fruit and vegetables as there was no electricity for freezers. I saw this same necessity in the forty years of raising my family of eleven children.

In this book I hope to encourage the reader to grow a garden, even just a small patch. Only then will the miracles of creation be known. There is nothing more exciting to me, than to see the tiny seed that one plants, sprout and grow to maturity. I also hope to encourage good stewardship of the soil. The earth is our mother where all food comes from. We must preserve the earth by using natural methods to sustain a balance. Then we can be sure our plants will be fed naturally by the soil itself.

The cycle of the four seasons gives us a good idea of what needs to be done. Life begins with a seed. It is planted, then sprouts and grows to full maturity. The dying of the plant, followed by the decay process of plant material completes the cycle of decomposition, putting back into the soil the exact substance the soil had. The cycle is simple to understand, so in reading this book, you will know my feeling of the necessity of the law and order of composting. Good nourishing food can be grown without the use of harmful chemicals. These pages of my journal will provide a source of alternatives to growing such a garden.

What we want is a living soil because living soil provides ecological balance required to grow healthy, disease-free plants. I believe we could study soil forever and still not understand the wealth we have by working with nature. Every day the miracle of growth takes place somewhere in the world.

To be successful in anything, one must set a goal, educate themselves, then firmly set a pattern of responsibilities to achieve that goal. Gardening is my passion. Educating people through seminars, tours of my garden, consulting and being a mentor to anyone who will listen are some of the rewarding duties I hope to perform in my senior years. In this book I will share with you the reader, the things I have learned.

ACKNOWLEDGEMENTS

I sincerely appreciate the many fine people who have encouraged me to put some of my experiences and knowledge of gardening into print.

Father Louis P. White, pastor and mentor in teaching me the skills of organic gardening.

My family and friends interested in providing personal and material assistance.

My daughters who encouraged me during hard times toward my goal of educating the readers. Their devoted time and creative services which were invaluable in this project.

My grandchildren for the drawings used as clip art.

Generose Bennett for her professional printing assistance, hard work, patience, dedication and converting the draft of this book into a fine manuscript.

Contents

Introduction i
Foreword iii
Acknowledgements iv

Chapter 1
  January 1
Chapter 2
  February 9
Chapter 3
  March 13
Chapter 4
  April 19
Chapter 5
  May 27
Chapter 6
  June 33
Chapter 7
  July 41
Chapter 8
  August 47
Chapter 9
  September 53
Chapter 10
  October 59
Chapter 11
  November 71
Chapter 12
  December 75
Companion Plants 81
Systems of Mineral Element Deficiency in Plants 86

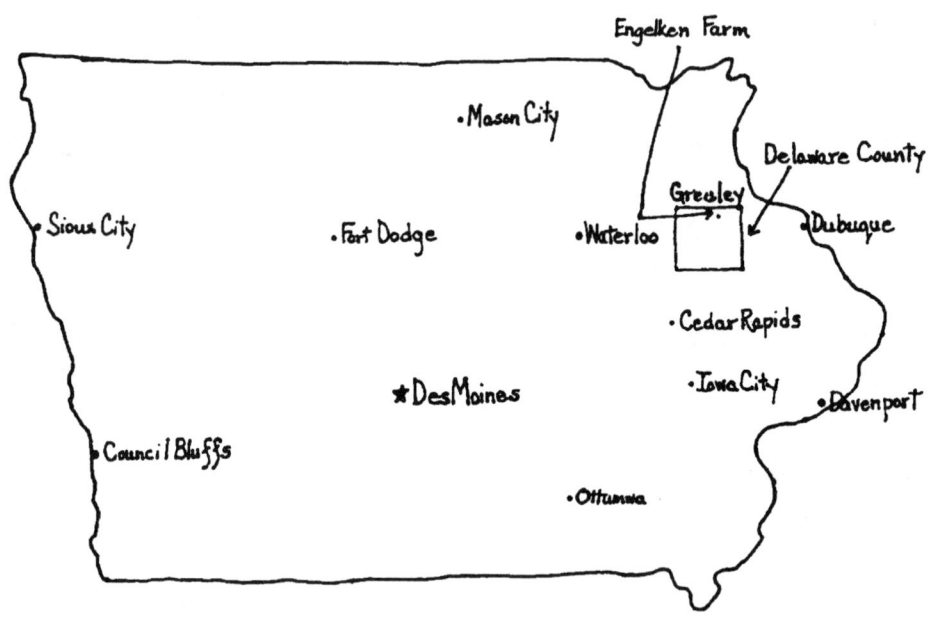

Iowa, heart of the cornbelt, where ten percent of the nation's food is grown.

JANUARY

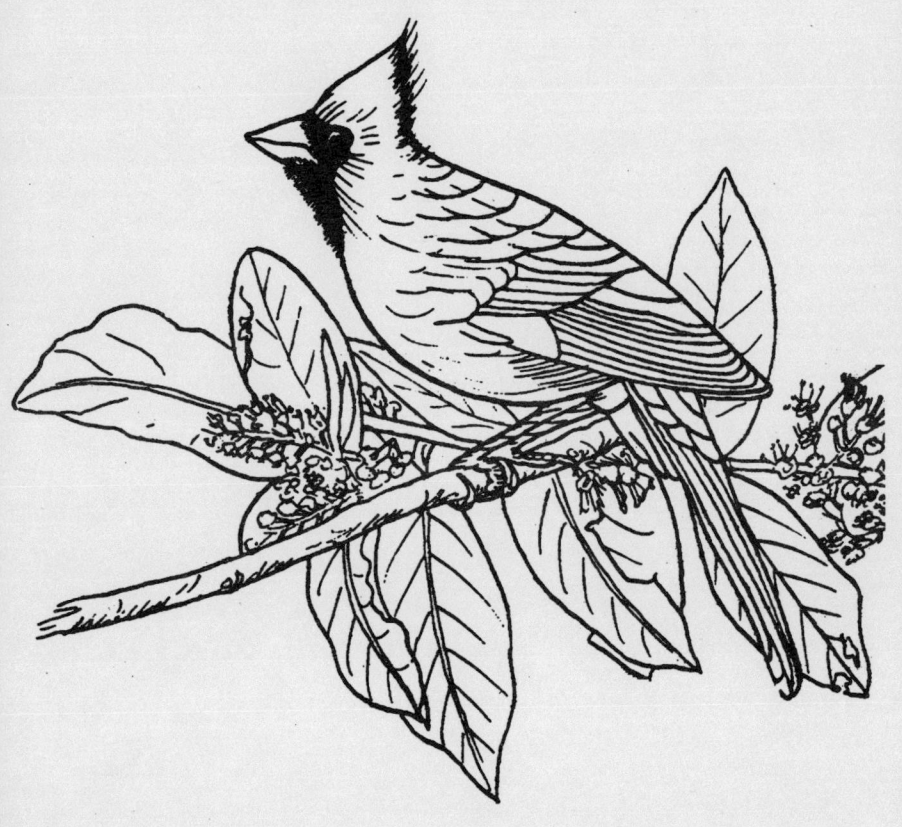

How pleasant to see the cardinal's brilliant flash of red against the winter snows! In the spring he makes cup-like nests in hedges.

JANUARY

Each January is a new year, a new beginning. Seed catalogs are already in the mail box. A catalog from every seed company means competition. This is a good time of the year to do a rating on how your garden has done for you in the past year. There is another good reason for taking that inventory of which varieties did well, which vegetable you liked the best, which was a good seller, and the keeping quality of potatoes, onions, squash and carrots. If you saved seed from your garden, check to see if the seeds germinate by placing a few in a flower pot. This way you will know if you need to order more seeds. Now plan your activities for the year. Will you have time to grow a small, medium or large garden? Usually the most depressing thing is when the weeds get ahead of you in the busy summer months. I'll be the first to admit that it takes time and you must set your priorities first. We tend to give up on gardening all together if nothing turns out right. This is why you must now set your mind to the garden size you can handle. Just remember, working the garden is beneficial for body and soul. It is a vigorous type of exercise and who of us does not need that?

I usually save my seed orders from one year to the next. If I did not like the seeds' performance I check them off. If you are starting out as a new gardener be sure to order the disease resistant seed and be sure it will grow in your climate zone. You can find this information in most seed catalogs. It is interesting to keep a record of the cost of seeds, the increase every year and the decrease of seeds to a packet. Hopefully this will motivate us to start saving our own seeds. If you keep saving seeds from the varieties you like your plants will be more resistant to

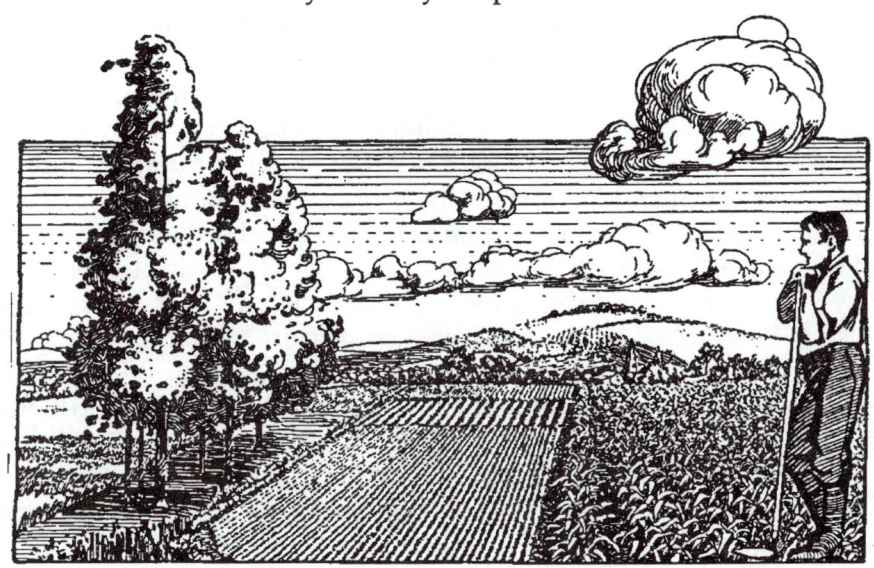

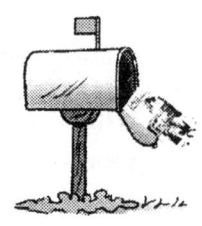
diseases. Hybrid-kept seeds will not perform the following year as well as they did the first. Join an organization like Seed Savers Exchange of Decorah, Iowa and learn how heirloom seeds are your best choice.

Even though the snow is covering the ground and winter winds are howling, you get a sense of spring coming soon when you leaf through these seed catalogs. There are always new varieties for us to try. But if you are firmly satisfied with the performance of last year's varieties, I see no reason to change. Make out your order, leave it around for a month, flip through the pages one more time to see if you've changed your mind, then put a reminder on your calendar to send the order out at least by the end of February. This is your genuine commitment.

Most seed catalogs are free. They have information on new seed introductions, starting seeds, maintenance, pest and disease control, harvesting dates and much more.

This time of year on a cold winter day, go to your library and get books to read on gardening. Make written notes of where you read articles of interest. Mental notes do not keep when times get busy as we tend to fall into our same old pattern of doing things. I keep a notebook of where I have read a super helping hint, or help in warding off insects the natural way. We must also remember not all recommendations work the same for every gardener.

Are we really aware of the money we save by growing our own food? Most of us would be reluctant to put a dollar value on our produce. I wish we could get into the habit of keeping a note pad in our cupboard door and mark down each jar of canned food, whether it is canned fruit, vegetable or juice. Let's not forget the root crops of potatoes, onions, carrots and turnips. Mark down the cost of these items just as if you were to buy them at the local supermarket. What about our frozen fruit and vegetables? The chickens we raised ourselves? We can be considered lucky if as a farmer or gardener we raise a variety of beef, pork, fish or chicken. Remember, all the food must come from the land.

We need to measure the real benefit from our gardens and fields, which is good health. Not only by eating the food do we maintain good health, but also we maintain the mental and spiritual values it gives. These savings achieved by growing a garden are the savings of spending a fortune on health clubs and exercising equipment to keep our bodies in shape. Not only do we spend hours weeding and tilling, but we also have the joy of watching the butterflies and birds and listening to the different songs of the birds. These melodies are the true vibration of frequencies in our universe. We can also watch the plants growing, changing their structure day by day. This should make us feel a part of the entire community of living things. We cannot put a price on values like these.

We need to choose from among the many conferences and seminars held this time of year for topics of particular interest and subjects that we would like to learn more about. Just to name a few sources of information, there is great help from vocational schools, Leopold Center, organic growers in many states and Natural Sustainable Agriculture. From these we can talk with people who have done some of their own research. Just attending these conferences is not enough. We must make a commitment to try some of the recommendations for our own gardens. It is easy to read or write about doing a job, but really doing it is what counts. Today there is an ample supply of literature in any library on raising your own food. Think of all these benefits in more ways than just having good food.

By now, in the middle of January, our house plants may need a boost. After growing all summer in your flower gardens it's like a prison to their roots when we put them in all those small containers. Not many nutrients are left in the soil in which you planted them. Let's give them a break and use an all natural fertilizer. A tablespoon of good compost to each potted plant is a start. My recipe for house plant fertilizer is in my December chapter. Fish emulsion is a good natural nitrogen source, but indoors it carries an odor that's not pleasant to breathe. Fish emulsion is a superior product that is 100% organic, made from fish containing 5% nitrogen, 5% phosphorus and 1.5% potassium, plus trace minerals to include selenium (2 p.p.m.) to revitalize soil and promote microbial growth and tilth. It can serve as a complete plant food or soil conditioner. Since it is 100% water soluble, it should be mixed with water before feeding plants. Each gallon of fish solubles represent 200 pounds of whole fish pulverized and stabilized. Fish meal is another way of processing the whole fish. It will take 30 to 60 days to break down so this is excellent to use in fall, or very early spring. This would be too slow a release for your indoor plants. We especially need to care for our greenhouse plants we received as gifts such as Poinsettias, Mums and Geraniums which were planted in soil-less mixes, commonly used at greenhouses in potting plants which contain a high amount of peat moss. If this mix gets too dry it becomes too difficult to let water through and the peat shrinks, causing a space between pot and soil-less mix. The water runs off the dry surface, down into the space and out of the bottom of the pot. It looks as though the pot is filled with water because it is running out the bottom, but the water is not actually soaking the roots, but starving the plant. To remedy this try watering slowly two or three times, waiting for half an hour in between to saturate the peat mix. If your water from the tap is chlorinated be sure to let it set in a container 24 hours before watering your plants. This chlorine will kill the micro-organisms in the soil and set your plants back from blooming.

Geraniums should be in bloom from now up to spring planting outdoors. With plenty of sunlight from a south or west window your geraniums in bloom should brighten up your days. A transplanted geranium grown in garden soil does better if allowed to dry out between waterings. A careful check on white flies must be observed at all times. If you notice them, a misting of insecticidial soap will usually take effect immediately. I then dust a light coating of diatomaceous earth on top of the soil in the flowerpot. This will kill the eggs in the soil where they hatch. When watering the minerals of the diatomaceous earth is food for the plant and the tiny diatons have sharp razor like edges to puncture the eggs of the insect.

The herbs you transplanted can be snipped off now for use in teas, soups and casseroles. My favorite herbs to bring indoors are lemon balm, parsley peppermint and chives. The lemon balm can be steeped in a container of water to deodorize your kitchen. What a nice lemony aroma. Parsley is used as a garnish, in salads and eaten raw or added to carrot juice. A combination of lemon balm, peppermint and comfrey makes a soothing hot tea sweetened with a little honey.

Inspect your stored bulbs and corms for signs of rotting or sprouting. This is caused by too much moisture, warmth or light. Remove all rotted roots to protect the remaining ones. Sprouted roots could be potted in a pot to replant in your garden next spring.

The perennial beds should be checked for signs of heaving. Cover any exposed roots with soil or a thick layer of mulch. Remove snow and ice from evergreens. Too much weight could break the branches. Also keep a watchful eye on young fruit trees. Rodents do a lot of damage to the tender young bark if any is exposed. This could kill your tree. Protect the trunk with chicken netting or tree wrap from your local hardware store. If a storm damaged any tree limbs prune those broken branches now to prevent further injury. If the mulch has thinned to where the soil is exposed around the fruit trees, bushes, vines or brambles, apply a fresh layer, holding it in place with boards or sticks. A wet, partly decomposed residue such as hay, straw, corn or beanstalks would be good material and would prevent blowing off. The secret of not having to do this tedious job in the winter is to use a thick enough mat in the fall. Always remember to keep mulch at least six to eight inches from the trunks of trees. Rodents such as mice like to make their nests close to tree trunks that are mulched.

Usually in our Zone 4 our feathered friends need a little help finding food. The Finch, Downey Woodpeckers, Cardinals and snow birds will be attracted to a feeder filled with their favorite food. Thistle seed and cracked sunflower hearts are favorites of the finch family. Their cheery voices seen to call one entire family to the feeder. Suet hung in mesh bags thrill the Woodpeckers and Cardinals. Another good idea is to make a suet cup of birdseed. As written in the November chapter, I melt down fat, then stir in a mixture of birdseed and pour it into Styrofoam cups. When the fat has hardened, break away the cup and tie it in a mesh bag on a tree limb close to a window so you can enjoy watching them feast. If at first the birds do not come, hang a colored ribbon nearby and they will check it out because it's something different in your yard.

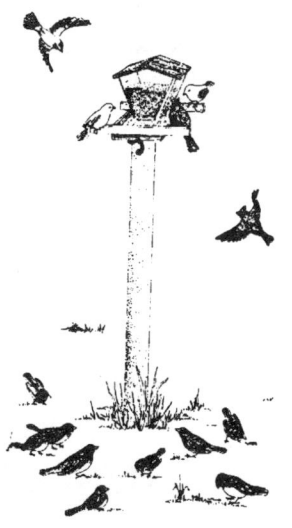
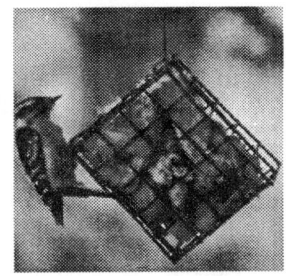
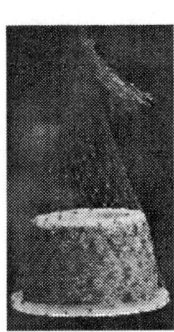
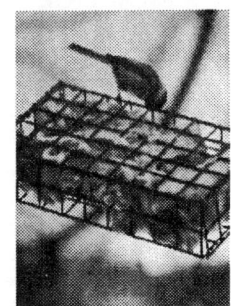

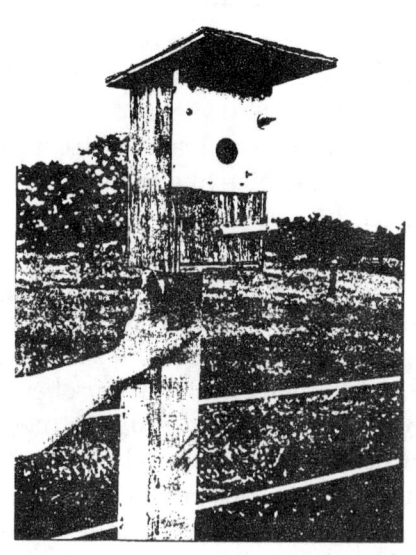
Sparrows and Starlings are disease carriers. Traps built especially for them when put at their resting zone can attract many birds. These traps are simple to build, any carpenter should be able to build one for you. The best time to trap sparrows is from June until the snow flies. Grain as bait with water attracts them when set under a tree or beside bushes that are their nesting place. Starlings are also a menace to song birds. They steal the eggs from the other nests which eliminates young birds. I know they are a supreme pest to my Martin colony. Their mean, long beaks crack the eggs in the nest, sometimes dropping them just below the Martin house. A good time to catch the Starling is when the snow has covered the ground. Traps baited with kitchen scraps is a good attraction for them. Setting this trap on the east side of a building or near shrubs where they perch on a cold winter day, sunning themselves, should attract many before spring arrives and their young are born.

This would be a good time to repair your bird houses or build new ones. Bluebird houses are easy to build and new Bluebird trails are being encouraged by our environmentalists. By helping nature along we can be assured of the balance being maintained.

BLUE BIRD HOUSE

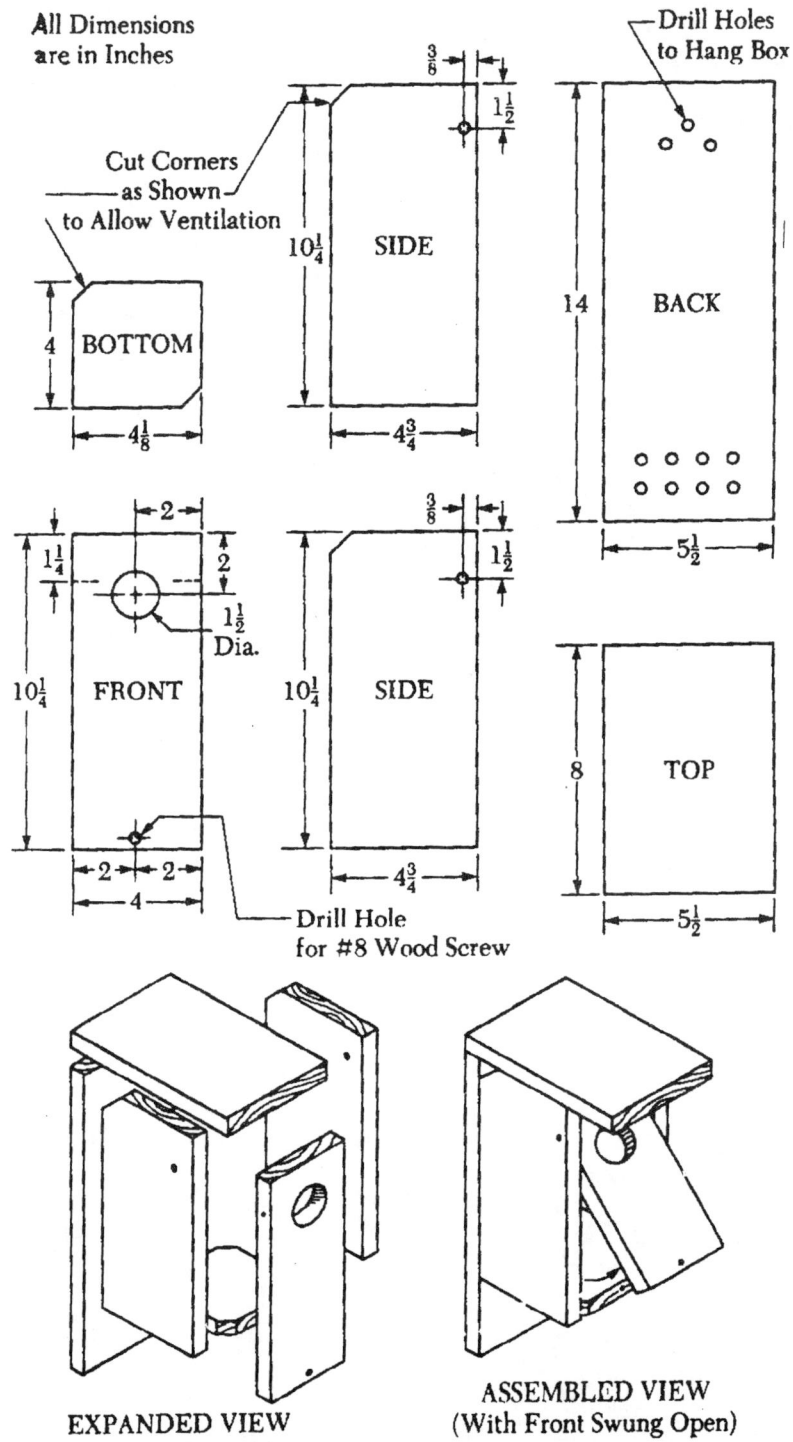

EXPANDED VIEW

ASSEMBLED VIEW
(With Front Swung Open)

FEBRUARY

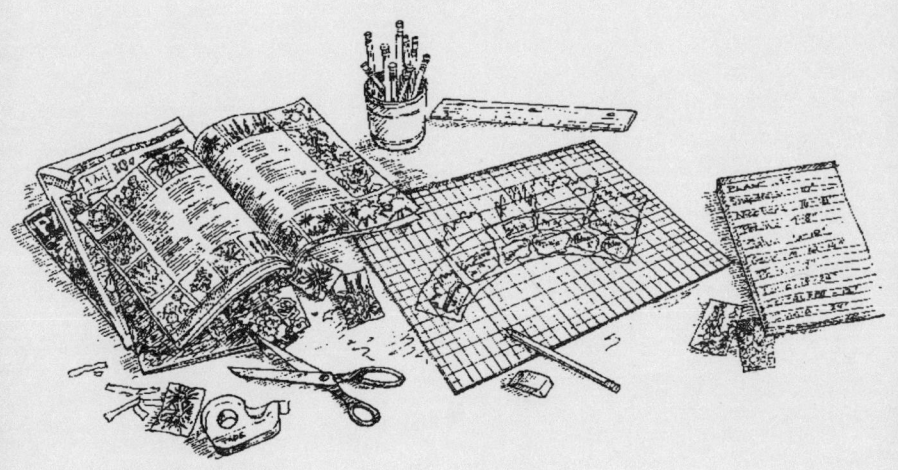

**To plant a garden is
to believe in tomorrow.**

FEBRUARY

It is a crisp winter day as we turn a new leaf of our calendar. February is the shortest month of the year, but that doesn't mean it's the least important month. On a brisk winter day you can see the birds coming to your feeders more regularly. The seeds and berries in the fields are now in short supply. The days are shorter, the nights are longer, and time spent by the fireplace or in a nice warm room with your favorite craft, whether it be knitting, quilting, crocheting or just the regular house chores, should be the rule of each day. There may be some leftover chores such as popcorn to be peeled or nuts to be cracked for your favorite recipe. Making these craft items can be your gifts to give throughout the year such as for weddings, birthdays, pen pals or bonuses for good grades in school. This then, is a part of your being self sustaining. Or maybe this is the time to learn a new hobby. Classes are held and can be attended to learn a new art. Trying something new is a real challenge, which requires cultivation of minds. Baking a new recipe to take to the next potluck meeting would be a nice gesture.

In the month of February we have a lot of celebrations, starting off with Ground Hog Day to predict the arrival of spring. Yes, we may still have six more weeks of winter, depending upon whether the ground hog saw his shadow or not. February second is about half way between the winter solstice and spring equinox, making it the year's four cross quarter days. We also honor two of our famous presidents in this short month, February 12th being Lincoln's birthday and Washington's birthday on the twenty second, with Valentine's Day in between. Serving appropriate meals on these days I can use the cherries, strawberries, beets and dried beans to bring out the color of red.

The magazines are having articles on starting seeds indoors, and how to grow them in nutrient soil. These are not excuses, but demands on getting involved again with soil and organic compounds. Reading articles like these give you ideas of how other gardeners handle their seedlings. In the full moon of February I slip my geraniums and other house plants brought in last fall from the flower garden. A full moon comes but once a month and in spite of winter still being here, spring will follow. In a dark colored jar I put water with a few drops of hydrogen peroxide, cut the slips with a sharp knife and insert them in this water until the roots appear. Then I transplant them into separate containers to move out to the flower bed. African Violets can be divided almost any time of the year. They tend to get root bound as they need a larger container. It's always nice to have a blooming plant to bring to a shut-in or a friend in a hospital to brighten up their day. African Violets can also be started with a leaf inserted in sand with a plastic bag covering the pot or tray, always watching that not too much moisture appears on the inside of the plastic. If this happens, remove it for an hour and then replace it again. February is the month to start rooting your sweet potato

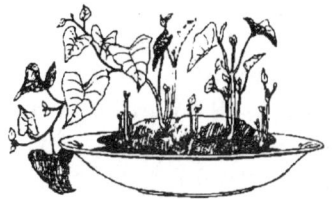 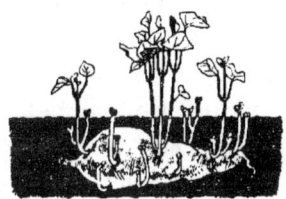 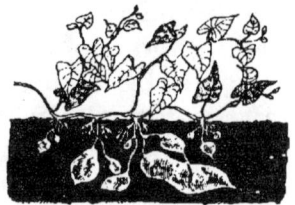

slips. Maybe you have sweet potatoes left from your garden. If not, purchase one from your grocery store and put in sand or a bowl or jar of water. This makes a lush vining house plant and you can use the slips to plant in you garden. They spread out as a crawling vine and need lightly sandy soil It is a member of the Morning Glory family brought over by Columbus from Central and South America to Spain. This sweet, delicate root can be used in many ways such as deep-fat fried, baked, stir-fried and pureed dishes.

Now is when we appreciate the soil and compost we brought in as extra dirt to repot our rooting slips and to start our seeds for transplants. One tablespoon or two of compost, worked into each flour pot, puts nutrients into soil to carry it through until its time to plant in your flower bed. Remember to go over your seed order you made out in January. Check it twice to see if you want to add or delete some of your gardening plans.

Let's learn a little about common herbs we take for granted:

PARSLEY: This is easy to grow and called "King of the Herbs". It grows prolifically and mixes with many foods. Parsley is a biennial so planting in early May and a late planting in July keeps two rows of it in fair condition through the winter. Use in soups, stews, juices and as a garnish. It grows well in a pot container and should be planted in a decorative container in the fall. Parsley is high in Vitamins A and C, also in iron and calcium

CHIVES: Chives are a member of the onion family, have a mild flavor and is good in cooked dishes, especially in stir-fry and steamed potatoes. Another good use is planting them among your roses to deter insects. The purple flower heads are an attraction in the flower bed, nectar for bees and beneficial insects and also can be used in dried flower arrangements. A gardener without a green thumb can grow chives. It is a very hardy plant.

DILL: This is a small hardy plant related to parsley, anise and caraway. It grows wild if not kept under cultivation. The dill plant is light green and when fully grown has an umbrella-like shape. Housewives use the seeds and tiny leaves for seasoning in pickled foods. Useful medicines are also made from dill. The umbrella shaped blossoms quickly turn into small flat oval seeds which change in color from the light green to brown. Seed in your flower garden for a nice contrast.

LEMON BALM: This highly scented herb comes from the mint family. Use as a room deodorizer by steeping a handful in a pot of boiling water. This is an uncanned lemon scent. The flowering herb makes a smooth tea blended with comfrey and peppermint, sweetened with honey. This plant, like most herbs, spreads profusely, so be careful where you plant it . Lemon balm fits nicely in your window sill garden. Snip off leaves to use but also dry extra from the garden for use in the winter months.

COMFREY: A super hardy plant which grows anywhere. Its priorities are two fold. The leaves are used in teas and snipped very, very fine in salads. The roots are used as a poultice for open sores. Comfrey is called the knitting herb because of its abilities to mend sprained ligaments. Leaves too are steeped and applied to open sores for fast healing. The leaves must be put in a cheese cloth wrap, then applied to the sore. Then use a bandage to keep the poultice in place. I think so very highly of this plant because it was introduced to our family in 1959 by Father Louie White, the Catholic priest who taught me everything I know about gardening. When he saw the sores on seven of our children and the open sore on my ankle he knew he had to help us with this plant. We had been to many doctors but received no help or cure. Father White said: "Rita, you must get those toxins out of your system before you can heal a sore with ointments." He brought me the leaves to steep for putting on the sores and also to drink as a tea. We then used the mashed roots he blended in his blender to apply on the worst sores. I could not believe how in three days time I could see the healing effects in the children's' skin. It was a cheap and simple remedy and will always have a place in my garden.

ALOE VERA: Who does not know of all the wonders of Aloe Vera? Medicinal use for burns, but now also the increase of knowledge in drinking the juice for perfect skin. These house plants are easily grown and a leaf is always handy for the unexpected burn from cooking. It takes very little care and multiplies quickly.

GARLIC: One herb everyone can grow. Knowing when to plant this bulb helps to grow a larger bulb. Planted in August, as I mentioned in my August chapter, will reward you with bulbs you can be proud to share with others, barter for trade or braid in a crafty arrangement to keep, sell or give as a gift. This herb also has many cleansing effects of our bodies. The medicinal values are too numerous to mention. Also used in seasoning foods and preserving foods. It does control high cholesterol and high blood pressure. Garlic tablets can be taken for this but would it not be better to eat what you have grown instead of something altered? Dried and hung in a cool, dry place, the bulbs will keep until fresh garlic can be used from your garden.

Does this give you an incentive to raise these common herbs? We're winding down to the last days of this short month, which is usually cold and stormy, but now and then there are sunny days to remind us that spring is not far off.

Primrose is the flower for the month of February. The primrose is grown in a shady spot of rich, moist loam. It can be started from seed which is planted in February in shallow pans or boxes. These plants can be transplanted in your flower bed in May. If protected well, they will over winter and flower the following spring. The primrose blooms in shades of violet and pinks, with the Amethyst the birthstone of February. This gem is purple or bluish-violet and resembles sincerity. What a nice way to end this month with the warm shades of both the flower and the stone.

MARCH

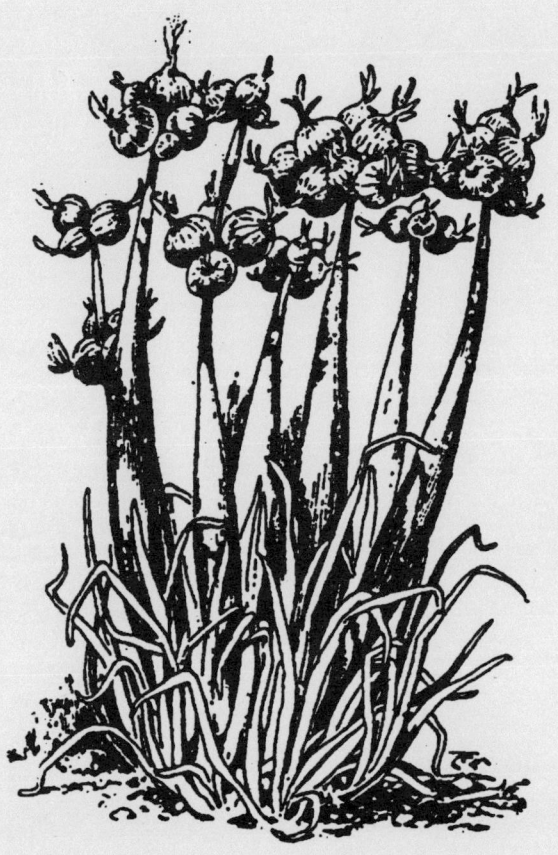

After the cover of snow is gone
these Egyptian onions come along.
The first greens of the year
makes me think spring is near.

MARCH

The popular belief is often heard if "March comes in like a lion it goes out like a lamb". The belief is that the first day is often stormy and the last day is mild. It is also believed that the first three days are unlucky, especially if it rains on those days, and they will have poor harvests.

This third month with thirty one days is the split between winter and spring. Spring in the northern half of the world begins with the vernal equinox which almost always occurs on March 21st. On this day the sun rises directly in the east and sets directly in the west, so that the length of the day is exactly equal to the length of the night. March can be both wintry and spring like, with blustery and windy days occurring as frequently as mild sunny days. As you continue to read these monthly chapters you will become more aware of what moon signs and an equinox is all about. They are very important in the makeup of our seasons so try to read and understand moon phases in the universe.

In the northern hemisphere many plants and animals awaken and come to life again during the month of March. The first pussy willows and wild flowers can be spotted in the protected woods. Hibernating animals like chipmunks and wood chucks leave their sleeping places. Wild geese and ducks can be heard honking their horns that they are back from the south. The first robin can be seen searching for food. Early songbirds appear in our sight. It is a month of no national holidays, but a celebration on St. Patrick's Day, March 17th, is observed by the Irish and the church. The clover leaf is a symbol of good luck and green symbolizes new growth in plants. Now we are serious about our seed catalog order. Send it out, commit yourself to growing at least the staple foods for your table. Spruce up your meals with the frozen fruits and vegetables in your freezer. Wouldn't a rhubarb pie be good for a change? Rhubarb is one of the first fruits to poke up through the surface of your garden. Finish up the peas you froze last June because more will be there to pick again. Prepare an all green meal for St. Patrick's Day, choosing from peas, beans, broccoli, green peppers, squash (yes, the green peeling), to the lighter shade of Chinese cabbage still stored in a second refrigerator. You may have green sprouts growing on your onions by now. Snip a little parsley and stir-fry all together for one great meal.

On the nicer days of March we must do the chore of trimming our trees and shrubs. Trim fruit trees first before they show any signs of budding out. This means before the sap begins to flow in the spring and when the trees are still dormant, but the wood is not frozen. Young trees are trained through light pruning. Pruning annually, cutting a small amount of wood each year, is much less of a shock to the tree. Branches cut correctly are done on a slant above the bud that is on the outside of the branch. Prune out older spurs because they begin to overcrowd the tree, refusing to let sunlight in. Maintain a horizontal growth pattern. Small fruits like grapes can be pruned in the month of March. You can trim grapes quite extensively. Cutting away some of the old wood makes room for the new. The vines may bleed sap but this does not harm the plants. Focus out the trunk of the vine. Keep the pencil thick canes with six inches between the nodes. These will bear the most fruit in this growing season. Presuming your grapes are trained on a 2 wire anchor, there should be branches on both sides of the trunk on the top and bottom wire. I leave three spurs on each branch that is left on the trunk. In the thirty four years of raising grapes I have never had a failure. These plants were given to me from Father Louie White's arbor of grapes. He was a true gentleman, always there with a helping hand. Now the big job in my garden is the everbearing red raspberry patch. The canes which bore fruit in the fall will have been cut down to waist high. Now all broken canes must be removed from the patch and burned. They cannot be composted or left in the patch. This is where we encourage the cane borer. The tedious job will pay off for you in nice big red juicy berries in June and September. The leaves and mulch you used last fall should show signs of decomposition, letting new shoots come through.

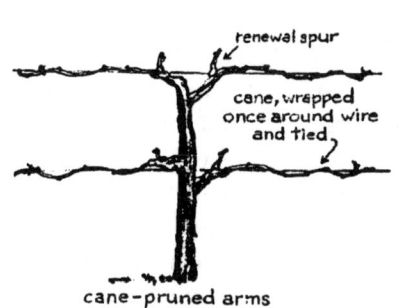

Any weeds should be pulled or hoed out to prevent further spreading in the patch. One reason for the mulch was to smother the weeds and the second reason was to hold the moisture. A dense growth of everbearers which grows two sets of canes is a thirsty bed. Remove all canes damaged by rodents and canes broken by wind. You have a rest now with this patch, but read my April chapter for more work for a bountiful harvest. Suckers on maple trees and shade trees can be cut off now. They like to grow close to the trunk of the tree. Any ornamental shrubs can also be trimmed, cutting away all dead wood and wrong way branches. Also, thin crowded centers of Forsythia, hydrangeas, redwood and weigelia. You can trim as much as one third of the shrub. They are so forgiving and regrowth is back in a couple of years. If you have a shrub you want to reshape you can cut it off completely and start over. The lilac bush cannot be trimmed in the spring. Only after flower heads have died do we trim the lilac. They are now setting flower heads.

Roses are next. Trim them two weeks before your last expected frost. Always use sharp shears to trim any branch, limb or shrub. Cut upright just above a bud. To shape a rose bush depends on your trimming inward or outward facing buds, always at an angle. It is still too early in my zone 4 to remove the mulch.

Another chore for March. For many gardeners it is seed starting time. For myself I do not start them indoors, but do have a perfect bed which is my flower bed on the south side of the house. I put square bales of hay or straw to hold out the wind and cold, and with wooden stakes I make a partition to separate beds. Plantings in late March are the cold crop plants such as cabbage, cauliflower, broccoli and head lettuce. A storm window laid across the top of the bales harnesses the heat from the sun and acts like a greenhouse. On cold nights I cover it with a blanket to hold in the heat. Tomatoes and egg plants are planted later. I treat these seeds with fish emulsion and seaweed solution...three tablespoons of each to one gallon of water. When these seeds grow they are immune to the cold and no hardening off needs to be done. I open the storm window on warmer days and this has been a real successful hot bed for me. Early in April the plants are growing nicely and can be transplanted by early May, still enough time for me to use this same bed to plant my flower garden. Compost made last fall is a must to get fast germination. The nitrogen from the fish emulsion gives it the boost it needs for a sure start. Seaweed is the insurance policy of many minerals to grow good plants. Don't be afraid to try different things. For some gardeners these methods may not work, but let me assure you it gets better as you go on. You will probably find as I have, that you keep learning new tricks each year, no matter how long you have been gardening.

Depending upon the weather, the sap is beginning to drip into buckets for the maple syrup. This is one job I have never done. I would like to be a student of a good sap drainer. I have been so fortunate to be able to barter my year's supply of maple syrup which is maybe the only reason I haven't tapped a tree.

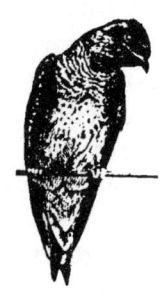

Purple Martins are first cousins of barn swallows. They winter over in Brazil and come to North America just to hatch their fledglings. As soon as spring arrives the martins also come, usually in late March and early April. The young fledglings of the previous year will look for their home as late as June, only to mark the nest for the following year. Their nests consist of small twigs and shiny leaves from the poplar tree. Your environment must be free of toxins to host a colony of martins. Each bird will consume 2,000 mosquitoes or 400 flying insects daily. Diatomacoues Earth must be dusted in the nest and on the fledglings to protect them from mites. The martins love to be worked with and enjoy people who give them credit for their busy days' work.

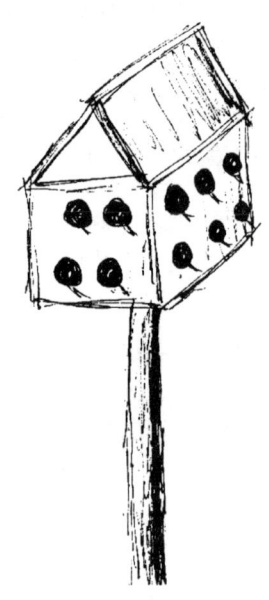

In the past years the purple martins came on the 25th of March. They arrive then because it's their natural instinct, but pattern changes in the universe influence weather conditions on the earth and it is too early because there are no flying insects. In these past two years we lost some of our early arrivals due to cold and starvation. Of course we had to open up the nesting boxes which makes a lot of work for housing only a few pair. The sparrows and starlings move in very fast. These nests need to be taken out every few days so when a scout comes their house is free of sparrow and starling nests. By next month more martins will move in and a strong colony can deter some of the sparrows. The frost is coming out of the soil so the gophers are already busy making mounds and damaging agricultural land. Gophers are very destructive, slightly heavier than a common rat. They have short legs and a broad, blunt head with small ears, small eyes and almost no neck. Its color varies from reddish brown to slate grey. The gopher's diet is grass, roots, nuts, buds, and farm vegetables, carrying its food in cheek pouches. The gopher digs with large, strong front claws and overhanging teeth. It rarely comes out of his burrow by day, but one can recognize them by a large mound of freshly dug dirt. This is a good time of year to poison them or set traps to capture them. They could destroy an entire field in one season. I use castor bean seed which I grow myself and dry in a warm place in the basement. These entire plants are poisonous and need to be burned when the frost has hit them. The clusters of bean seed can be podded and stored in a marked container out of reach of children. Sometimes I cut up potatoes in small pieces and mix them with copper sulfate purchased from a local hardware store. You can see the chipmunk holes as you walk the land and now is a good time to drop a poison pellet in their runway. These small rodents will steal your garden peas when they are almost ready to pick. Farm cats do come in handy at this time of year. A good mouser can be patient and wait for this little chipmunk to come out from his burrow. Hawks occasionally will snatch one as he flies over the fields. To do a good job of controlling these rodents you need to check the garden every morning.

The best fertilizer on the land is the farmer's foot prints. This also holds true for the gardener. To see the plants as they mature makes you a partner of that soil. Lawn raking can begin now whenever there is a little sunshine. The fresh air is a health tonic and assures you of warmer weather to come.

In March people begin to look for the first robin, a sign of spring. Early songbirds appear. The flower of March is the violet with heart shaped leaves forming a five petal flower. Each flower grows gracefully on a slender stalk. There are white and yellow varieties, but blue and purple varieties are the worlds' favorites. The gem of March is bloodstone.

Proper wasys to prune roses

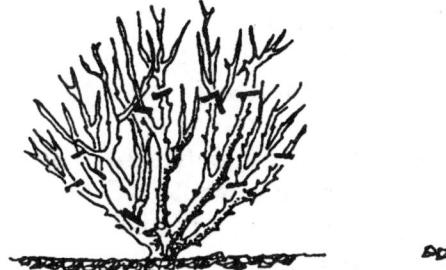 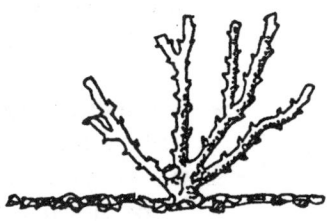

Remove deadwood, weak and twiggy branches, any crossed branches.

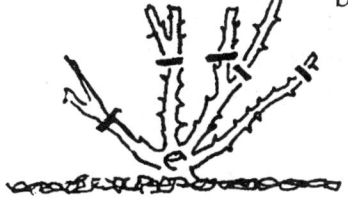 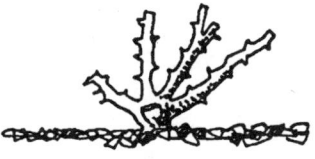

In cold climates, reduce bush to half the size it was in the fall.

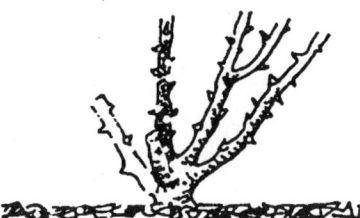 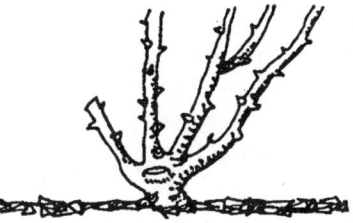

Don't leave a stub when cutting off a cane at the bud union.

ELUSIVE SPRING

Sprintime plays her little game
Of peekaboo each year.
Now you see her; now you don't —
When next will she appear?

She's warm; she's cold; she's in between.
She's never what you guessed!
You start your day with coats and hats;
By noon you're overdressed.

When pleasant days arrive at last,
You grab your gardening hoe.
"Gotcha!" says elusive spring.
"Next week, I'm sending snow!"

APRIL

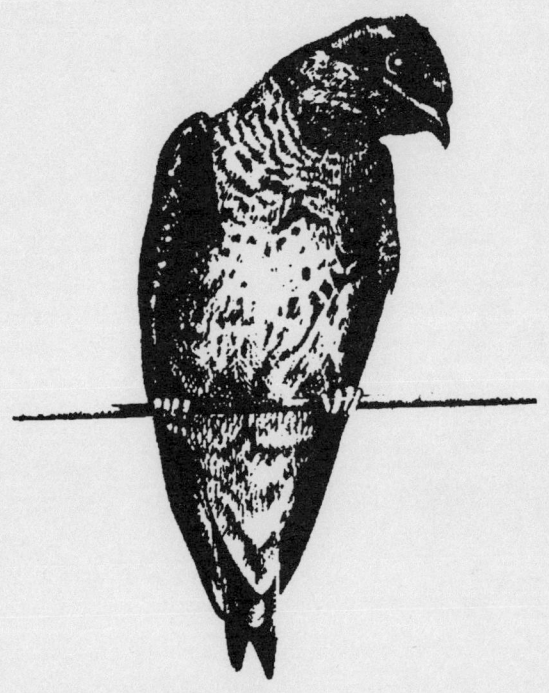

The best way to boost the nesting success of martins is to monitor their nests weekly.

APRIL

You have now read the entire book! No, not really...only April Fools Day has appeared! This month's saying is April showers bring May flowers. You will see signs of many new shoots coming up everywhere. And our seed order has arrived so it is serious planning of what to plant when. My hot-bed greenhouse is all sprouted and the sun is getting stronger to provide light and warmth to the growing plants.

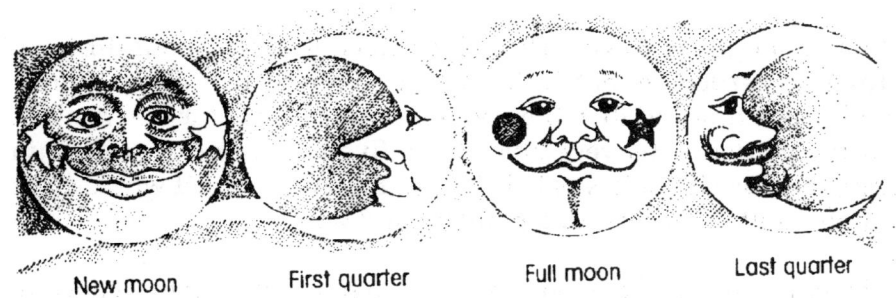

New moon   First quarter   Full moon   Last quarter

The earth in its passage about the sun passes the latter two thirds of one sign and the first one third of the next sign each month. The moon revolves to circle the earth once in 29½ days, passing through all the signs. The sun reaches the meridian at twelve o'clock four times a year. April 15, June 14th, September 1st and December 25th. The Lyrids peak around April 22nd which in 1993 is around New Moon, so moonlight will not hamper observations. Watch for at least five to ten "shooting stars" an hour from high in the sky at around midnight for several nights. It would be wise to get your almanac now if you haven't done so already. You will need it to follow me in my garden chores.

This month of April always brings memories each year. In 1959 it was our first introduction of growing foods without chemicals. We had moved seventeen miles west of the farm where we were harmed by custom spraying of harsh chemicals. Father Louie White would come each day to encourage us to listen to his message. He had been successfully growing a garden the natural way on the parish grounds for many years. His main concern was restoring the health of our family. The restless children and our nerves all stressed was easy to see as he visited us. His main message was, grow all your own food with natural supplements, but of more immediate importance was to get rid of all white sugar, white flour and all preserved foods. This meant all prepared mixes, canned foods and cold cereals. I knew he really was a person wanting to help. Just starting the garden season he brought me a lot of different plants and seeds he had saved from his garden and volunteered plants that came up in his compost heap.

We set out fruit trees, grapes, red raspberries and a long row of popular trees. These were fast growing and had two main purposes. One was the oxygen cleansing effect in the air, the other for bird habitat. Then in the fall these leaves all fell into my raspberry patch for mulch. I found out as I picked the raspberries the popular trees grown on the east side of the patch provided shade long into the forenoon, making the task a pleasant one.

I had a long way to go. There was much to learn about this new approach to gardening, but Father White's fatherly care of the parish grounds came first and then there was still ample time for him to assist me in my garden. His vegetables were five to seven days earlier in ripening because his soil was in balance. He assured me I would have the same results. I just needed patience and time.

The soil is where all the food comes from so this is your first concern, and the right time of the year to prepare the soil. Your decisions will be determined by the amount of toxins in your soil. For many, a soil test may be necessary. It would be a sure way of knowing what to apply. A soil P-H of seven is a good balance, but may not be the complete answer. In a garden there are many varieties of crops grown where some acid soils are necessary. Blueberries need an acid soil. Potatoes lean to an acid soil. This is where those seminars and conferences that I suggested you attend in February and March were so very important. One may never understand your soil completely because as a plant grows it takes from the soil and may only replace that nutrient in its decay process. This is why I am an advocate of composting. We can read in many books the value of compost. It adds humus to the soil which turns into organic matter through decomposition, therefore feeding all the micro-organisms in the top six inches of the soil where all roots begin to develop. I guess I can truthfully say that if compost is made correctly with the Bio-Dynamic Starter developed by Dr. Ehrenfried E. Pfeiffer, and applied each spring or fall, the balance of your soil will come faster than from any other method. Compost made with the 55 strains of beneficial micro-organisms is ready to attach the eggs of the bad bacteria living in the soil as soon as your soil reaches 50 degrees. This compost will never burn your plant roots. It will enhance germination because of the humus content it holds so our early rains can be absorbed in the top four to six inches of the soil.

The self education by reading about soil is so very important and many books are printed today for the knowledge of understanding soil structure.

Father White introduced us to Silent Spring by Rachel Carson, Dr. Albrecth, a soil scientist from Missouri, the practice of Rudolf Steiner and Dr. Ehrenfried Pfeiffer. Even today these pioneers' names come up in every natural fertilizers conference. We will never know all there is to know about soil because of weather patterns changing, and our ever changing environment. Our task is to learn to become stewards of the soil.

We must not work our soils too wet in early spring. This tends to harden the soil and your task of raising a garden can be hindered. My first job is to turn under the green manure of wheat I sowed last fall. Depending upon its growth because of weather, I may need to mow it off first. Then rototill into the soil, and a period of four to five days is needed to break that down. The soil will be humus and soft under the wheat roots. If there is enough bacteria in the soil this green manure should decompose easily.

Now we are ready to start seeding the very early crops. With the garden plan we put down on paper as we made out our seed order, it should be easy for us to do our planting. Companion planting does help but is not always necessary.

Peas planted as early as possible will yield the best. Planting two or three different varieties help stagger your pickings. Depending upon how you will preserve them will play an important part in choosing the right variety. Little Marvel has been a consistent early pea for me. Green Arrow has been another favorite. Always plant a few more than you need yourself, some for those you care and some to share. You'll enjoy eating them fresh, right from the pod, sneaking them as you hoe or walk through your garden. I freeze most of my peas as they are a real treat all winter long.

Onion plants do best if planted early this month. Again, this is the reason for your early seed order. The plants usually are not in the stores yet so a week makes a real difference. They can even stand a light frost or snow cover, which is also true of early planted peas.

We are so excited about planting seeds...to watch them sprout and grow into edible food. The only vegetable we must not plant early are the beans. They are very susceptible to early frosts. In my zone 4 it is too early for tomato and green pepper plants, but the cold crops can be transplanted and covered for protection. I use the plastic milk jugs with the bottoms cut out and lids removed. This creates a hot bed effect. One needs to push the jug into the soil to prevent the wind from blowing them away. Setting a few each of cabbage, cauliflower, broccoli and kohlrabi gives you an early start in eating fresh vegetables from your garden. The seeds of all of these can be planted, but only when the moon phase is right. Remember what I keep saying; there is a real reason for the moon, sun and stars. The root crops are always planted in the dark of the moon and the above ground crops in the light of the moon. Try to plant a day after this moon sign change which gives a more accurate planting success. Yes, I agree you do need an almanac to follow and for a bonus you can read a lot of hints and suggestions.

Work up only the amount of soil you intend to plant. The wind and rain has a tendency to erode the fine earth. We must save all the top soil available.

The onion sets can also be planted. I use the old time multiplier onions. I never have to buy sets. With these you plant one set and get five or six onions to eat. Always save enough to let die back to dig in the fall. This is another savings we fail to consider in growing a garden. What is more refreshing than green onions early in May? And do we really know the value of the onion? A lowly plant, but it's high in Vitamin C. Its pungency comes from volatile sulfur compounds that are released by an enzyme when the skin is damaged. Much more than anything else, the genetics of the plant influences the sulfur content. Many varieties are available, all depending upon what you demand of the eating quality.

Now the buds are beginning to show on the berry bushes and fruit trees, grapes and bushes. This time of the year is indeed a busy one. I faithfully mist all plants, trees and bushes with a bath of fish emulsion. A pump sprayer works well, but I have used a sprayer attached to a hose with the required strength calculated out according to the pressure that is connected on your garden hose. I give this bath of fish emulsion (3 tablespoons to 1 gallon of water) three times to all plants before their bloom stage. Be sure to read the labels of your fish emulsion, refraining from any that contains chlorine to take away odor. The chlorine will kill live bacteria and destroy the beneficial micro organisms in your soil. Again, this misting must be done early in the morning or after sunset. This is the only time the pores of the plant can absorb the treatment.

The time to take the mulch from your roses will depend upon your frost dates. In a well protected area you can do that chore this month. Be sure to add some compost to the roots, add a thin layer of mulch to conserve moisture. A misting of fish emulsion will guarantee a healthy plant with glossy dark green leaves before buds set.

As early as possible when the weather warms up, April is the time to use our dormant oil spray on the trees. A dormant oil spray is applied to orchard trees before any of the buds open. Some gardeners use a dormant oil spray on shrubs and evergreens every spring, but it's rarely necessary if these plants have been grown organically a number of years. Fruit trees have many enemies and dormant spraying is necessary. In early spring insects hatch from eggs laid on plants and in protective cocoons on twigs and branches. The dormant oil seals over these egg cases, preventing them from hatching. One can purchase a miscible oil in your garden supply center, or make your own as follows:

½ C. fish emulsion   1 C. liquid detergent
½ C. mineral oil

Stir or shake vigorously to combine all ingredients. Mix this solution in 1 gallon of water. Spray the entire tree, shrub or evergreen at one time so as not to allow some insects to survive.

After this treatment a beneficial insect should be in place to take over. If you are not familiar with the beneficial insects you may have to order these to incorporate them into your garden and yard. The tricogamma, praying mantis and lady bugs are very important. Spacing these hatches will be of great value because not all insects hatch at the

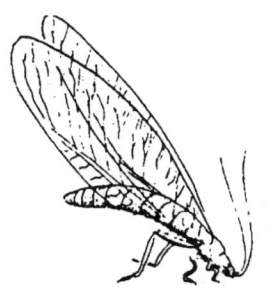

Green Lacewing

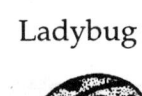

Ladybug

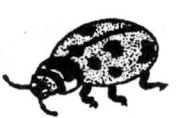

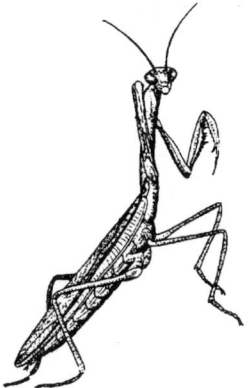

Praying Mantis

same time. It is a relief for me to notice these beneficial insects for that tells me they will control and keep the insect population in balance.

The rock garden perennials should be peeking through the soil along with spring flowers like peonies, phlox, corrabelles, johnny jump ups and primrose. Leaving the mulch around these plants protects the plants and the nests of lady bugs still nestled in their winter homes. I know it's the time when everyone wants every leaf picked up in their yards and along foundations but be aware of the balance you will destroy if colonies of beneficial insects are under this for winter protection. Until the destructive bugs attack your area there is nothing for the beneficial insect to eat. We must remember that both species are each others' keepers.

We as gardeners flow very easily through this month. What does not get done in April always can be finished in May. This is our insurance policy for weathering the winter.

Dandelions are springing up everywhere. As a child it was the first flower stem we brought to our mother. Innocent as we were, we truly loved the flower. I also knew butterflies would come to visit the flower. I would sneak into the cellar to get an odd jar and sit very quietly until the butterfly would land on a yellow dandelion flower. Then I would catch it in my jar, just long enough to study its color, then let it fly away again. I find myself still catching butterflies and insects to learn about their benefits to nature.

This month has gone by fast with many chores still to be done. The garden plan I drew out in March has helped to guide me to what comes next. The sun is getting stronger and the days longer, assuring me of the May flowers promised by the April showers. The long wait for winter to disappear makes April and May the most refreshing of months.

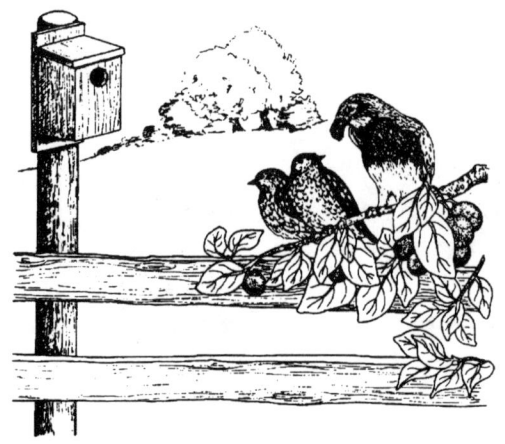

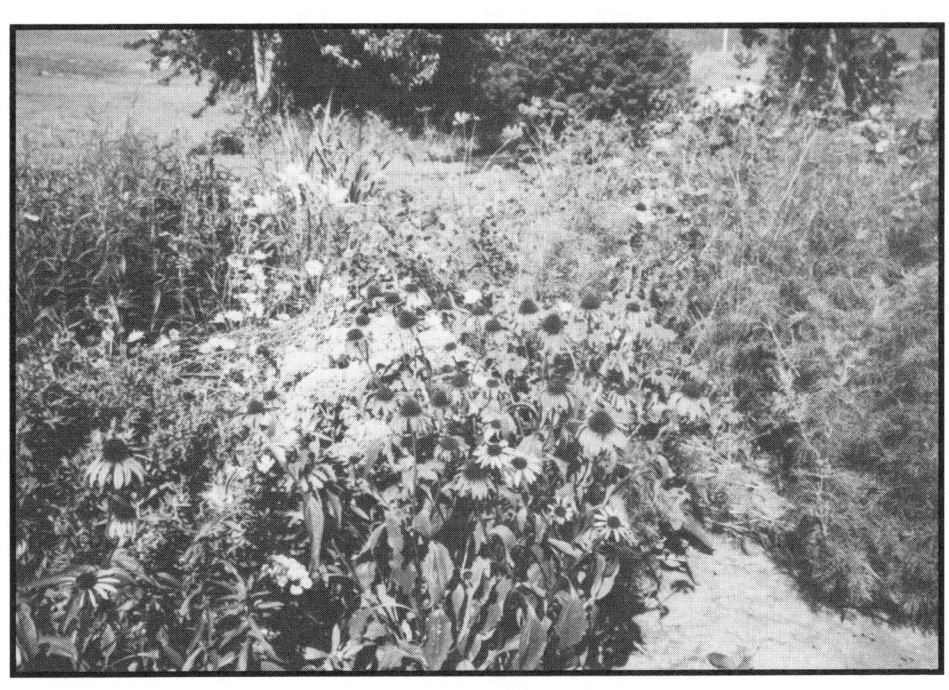
Perennials all blooming at different times.

April was the second month in the early Roman calendar, but it became the fourth month when Julius Caesar established the Julian calendar in 46 B.C. April in Latin means to open.

On the first day of April children and grown ups play jokes on one another. Arbor Day is a day for planting trees and is observed on various April days. Easter nearly always falls in April and brings with it other Christian religious celebrations such as Palm Sunday, Holy Week and Good Friday.

April is mainly a sowing time on many northern farms. Yet in some parts of the world it could be grain harvest time. The flowers of April are the sweet pea and the daisy. The birthstone is the diamond, the most costly jewel in the world. The size of diamonds are determined by their weight in carats.

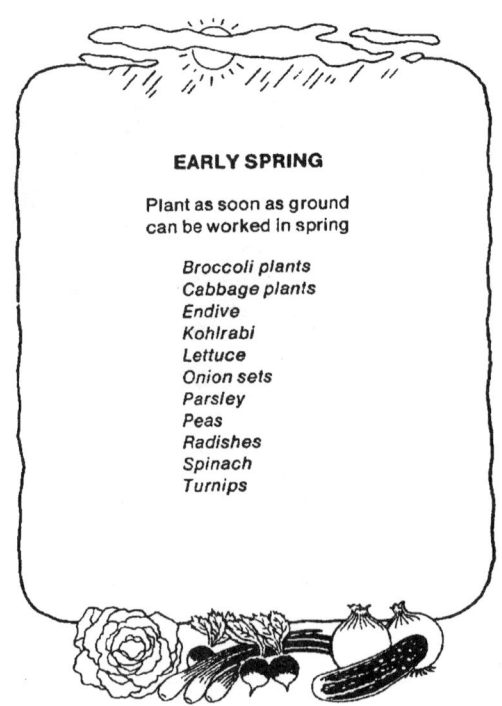

EARLY SPRING

Plant as soon as ground can be worked in spring

Broccoli plants
Cabbage plants
Endive
Kohlrabi
Lettuce
Onion sets
Parsley
Peas
Radishes
Spinach
Turnips

MAY

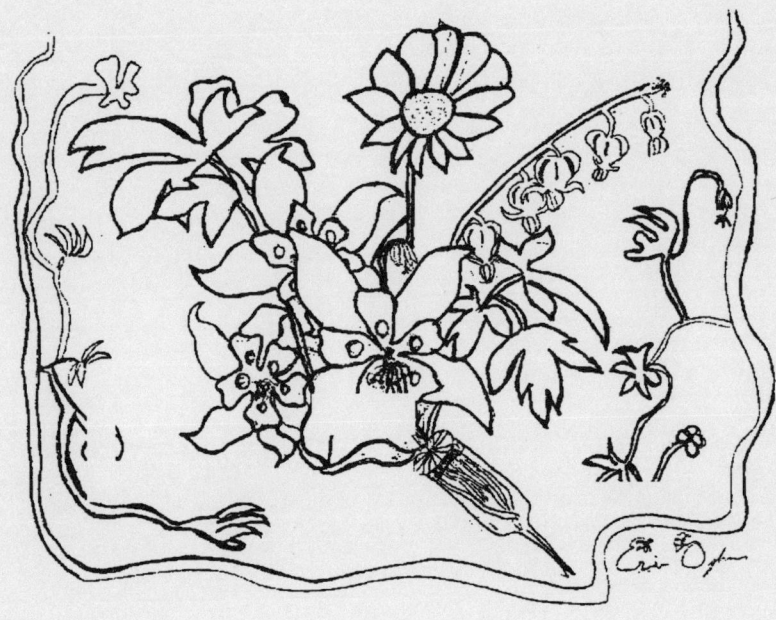

I love to watch the miracle when blossoms bud and grow. I am nearer to God in my garden than anywhere else I know.

MAY

May is one of the most beautiful months of the year in the northern temperature zone. The winter snow and ice has melted and the summer's intense heat has not yet begun.

We are starting off the month with May Day by displaying all sorts of May baskets. Whether they are woven, crocheted or assembled from flowers grown in the woods, it is the first day of celebration. Things are happening! The trees are showing signs of green, grass is a welcome site, wild plants are in bloom. Many birds have already built their nests and mother birds are sitting on the eggs soon to hatch.

I know we are all busy this month with timely chores, but each week now, we must remove sparrow and starling nests from the martin houses. Should there be a nest built in the martins' home when they arrive, they will move on and we don't want that to happen. Most of last year's pairs will come back so our efforts to encourage another scout to bring his partner to be a member of our colony is most important now. Failure to do this is why most colony owners never increase their pairs.

The May apple is an American plant belonging to the barberry family. This grows wild in wooded areas in large groups or colonies. The large leaves have five to seven lobes which look like umbrellas. They usually grow in pairs on a stem one foot high, then the white flower grows on a short stem in the form of a stalk which is two inches wide. A yellow fruit forms which resembles a lemon and has a sweet taste. The fruits are used as preserves. A delicious treat...try some!

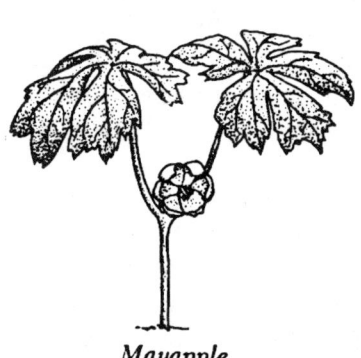
Mayapple

The root of the May apple contains podophyllin, a poisonous substance, but when dried it is used in making a cathartic drug which is a laxative. An interesting insect called the May Fly is a dainty insect with lacy wings and a slender tail. They are often called Day Flies because of their short lives. They do not eat or have stomachs, thus they are a food for fish. They are common in spring but can occur in late fall.

We are serious now about our planting schedule. Hopefully our onions and peas are already planted. All cold crops can now be planted in garden rows for future transplanting. The many varieties of lettuce need to be planted now. Green leaves of all perennials should be protruding from their winter home. This is the time to give all budding plants and bushes their bath of fish emulsion. Three tablespoons to one gallon of water is the recommended portion to use. We use this on our strawberry bed, our raspberry canes, the grape vines, the fruit trees, the flower beds, and our not-to-forget evergreens. The evergreens may be showing signs of stress from winter wind burn. We must nurse these along by giving them a shot of nitrogen-yes, fish emulsion. Look for the mite damage that could be occurring. They eat the juice of the needles, making them yellow, and then they disappear, leaving only a dry stem. A coating of diatomacoues earth on a quiet evening will kill those mites. Dust dry at sunset and leave on the branches a few days. Usually a yew will not need additional fertilizer but only a good mulch in the fall so the roots can be protected. These yews can be trimmed in May which will let the remaining plant use the nutrients it needs from the soil. For a beginner just planting rootstock, be sure to remove the burlap wrapping because this prevents the new roots from taking hold in the soil A good amount of well made compost is an absolute must to get roots started. Watering with fish emulsion treated water with an additional ingredient of sea kelp is good insurance of a healthy plant. The same solution, which is three tablespoons each of fish emulsion and sea kelp to one gallon of water, will be your guarantee.

Watch for our moon signs when planting your vegetables. I must tell you that it does make a difference. If you are not a believer of moon planting signs, just do your own research. You will know only if you do it for your own benefit. Plant a few radish seeds for thirty days, keeping an accurate record of planting dates to prove to yourself that the dark of the moon grows root crops, the light of the moon foliage. You can see and learn from the results of your own research.

All your mulches should be removed from roses by now and clean compost and a half cup of bone meal per bush should be fed to them. This is lightly worked into the top soil. Then clean mulch should be applied to hold moisture and prevent the rain drops that splash on the dirt which provides the spores of black spot. Other mulches can be left for protection but most will be decomposed to add nutrients to the soil.

Some of the earlier crops are planted and it is now time to expand planting space for later crops. Therefore I like to work up only the area where I will be planting in my garden. The wheat that was sowed as a green manure crop is now growing profusely and needs to be mowed off again. Tilling two days after mowing should give you a rich loam soil. Some roots may be visible but it's good organic matter which will decompose and should be no problem to the gardener. Usually no weeds will grow where wheat was planted and turned under.

It is very helpful if we made our garden plan on paper in March and April when we were ordering our seeds. That makes it easier to get right to planting. We should have studied our companion planting chart. A good rule of thumb is what tastes good together grows well together. The onion family, like leeks, garlic and chives, are good repellents scattered throughout the garden. Marigolds and nasturtium are also good repellents. It makes a splash of color throughout the vegetables when sparsely set between the cabbage, broccoli and cauliflower plants.

Companion planting is only a hired hand. You need a good soil structure and balance. The top six inches of soil, where the organic matter is located, is the most important. Aeration by earth worms is the greatest asset to a garden. If your soil is depleted of earthworms you may have to find a good source to order them and incorporate them in your soil. Doing this is not a hard chore. When you get your worms, dig holes one foot deep and one foot in diameter. Fill each hole with some good soil, compost, worms and worm food. Yes, worms need food too. A good selection is cornmeal, oatmeal and a little powdered milk. Now you have a happy colony of earthworms. They will breed fast and spread out, helping your entire garden.

All plants are growing fast and it's a pleasure to walk through the yard and garden, watching each one unfold into a mature living substance. Do not forget to capture some of this excitement by taking photos of your handiwork to pass on to the next generation. The saying is, a picture is worth a thousand words.

When I was a child we had a church service in May where we marched in a procession from the church to the cemetery. The girls in grades one through eight would carry baskets of flower petals and drop a few as we marched to three chapels in the cemetery. Each year as the peonies open I always think about those days of prayer and devotion.

We also have Mothers Day in May. A flower gift from our own garden can mean so much to our mothers.

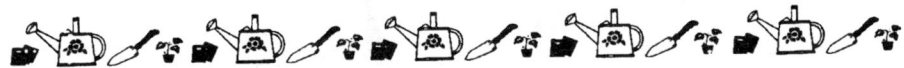

Our first holiday, Memorial Day, also comes on one of the last days of May. We can show honor to the generation before us and our loved ones who fought for our freedom by decorating their graves with flowers. Our presence also shows respect for those who cared enough in their lifetime so that we can reap their benefits.

We can plant our bulbs of gladiolas, dahlias, day lilies and cannas. Breaking each corm apart will assure you of a larger bloom. This will also give you a larger supply for next year's planting. Or you may want to offer some for sale or trade with other gardeners for a flower you do not have. These bulbs usually do not take any special care other than a supply of compost over the bulbs and water to make them take root.

Now too, is the time to hang the milk jugs in your fruit trees. I save my juice from pickles, beets and relishes to use as a base of liquid in these jugs. Cut a three inch hole on one side of the jug opposite the handle. Use a nylon tie to hang the jug on a tree branch. Use a vinegar, water and sugar mixture to attract flying moths which will mature into a worm. The exact mixture is not really important...just the scent of the vinegar and sugar will make the moths hungry. Of course they will then drown in the liquid. I put the cap on the jug so they are captured in the jug. You will be surprised at how many moths you will attract. You may need to change this liquid two or three times a year. The lady bugs or lace wings are not attracted to this solution because it's not their survival food.

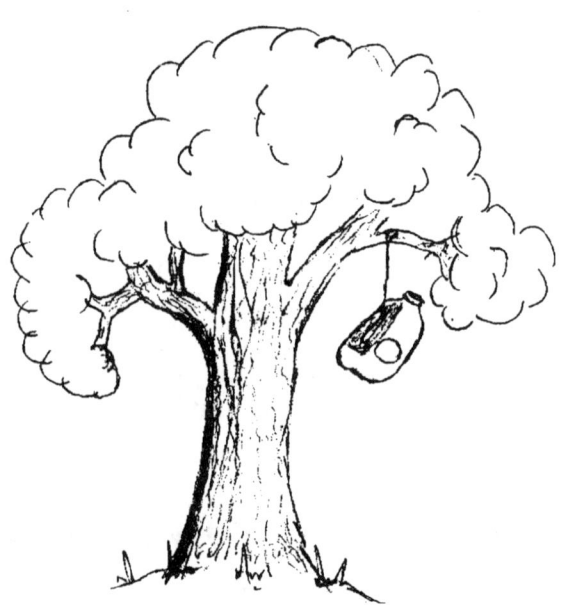

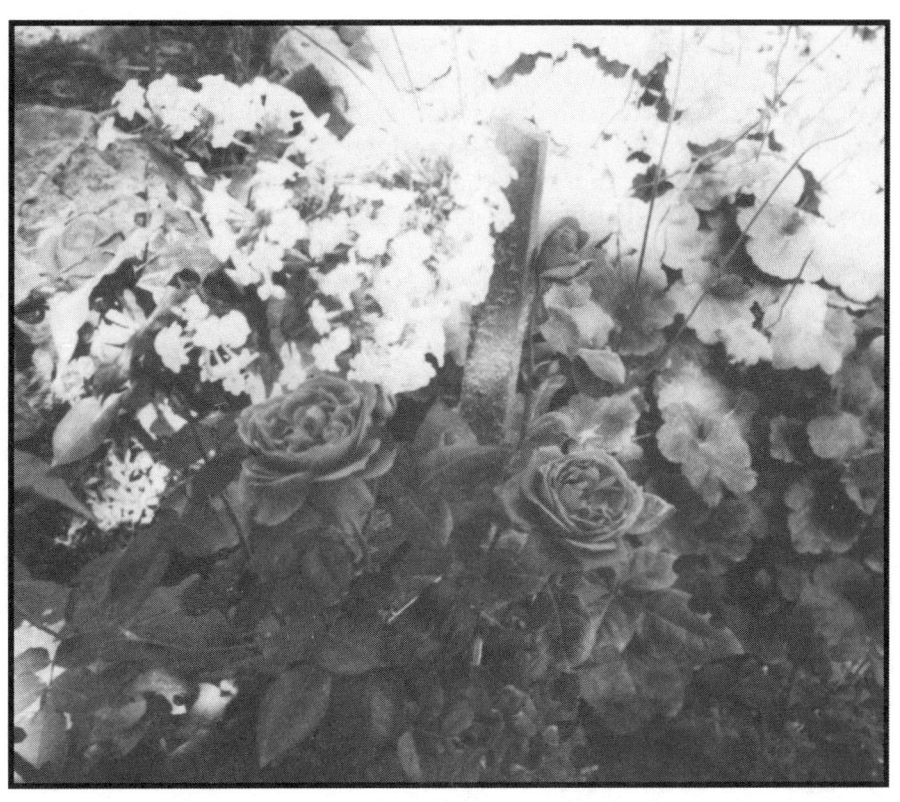

Disease free roses foliar fed with fish emulsion

Transplanting can take place at the end of this month. Some protection will still be needed in Zone 4 where I live. A late frost could set your plants back. When a plant is stressed it seems hard to bring it to full maturity.

The vine crops can also be planted. These plants need special care, watching very carefully for the striped cucumber beetle. Natural controls are covering with cheese cloth, use of dusting with distomacoues earth or insecticidal soap sprays. The insect predators are various soldier beetles. The golden or dull orange with black markings on the wings, a black head, soft body called the leather wing soldier beetle feeds on grasshopper eggs, cucumber beetle and various caterpillars. The secret is not to allow the egg masses to hatch. Planting radish seeds in the hill is another deterrent. The eggs are laid near the root and come up through the ground close to the stem of the plant. Putting one fourth cup of wood ashes in the hill when you plant your seeds is another helpful hint.

From now on a daily walk is very important to keep a watchful eye on insect damage and getting a head start on their control. Remember the old saying, "a stitch in time saves nine".

The Hawthorn and the Lily of the Valley are the flowers of the month and were used to trim the May pole by the Romans. The beautiful bell shaped flower is pure white and hangs down in a long cluster along a tender stem. It is famous for its delightful fragrance, one of the first flowers to bloom.

Emerald, being the birthstone of May, is so appropriate, being green. This stone is the next best thing to having a diamond.

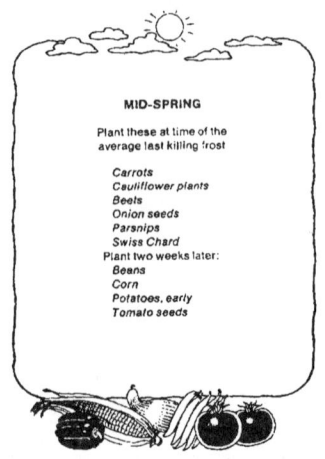

MID-SPRING

Plant these at time of the average last killing frost

Carrots
Cauliflower plants
Beets
Onion seeds
Parsnips
Swiss Chard

Plant two weeks later:
Beans
Corn
Potatoes, early
Tomato seeds

JUNE

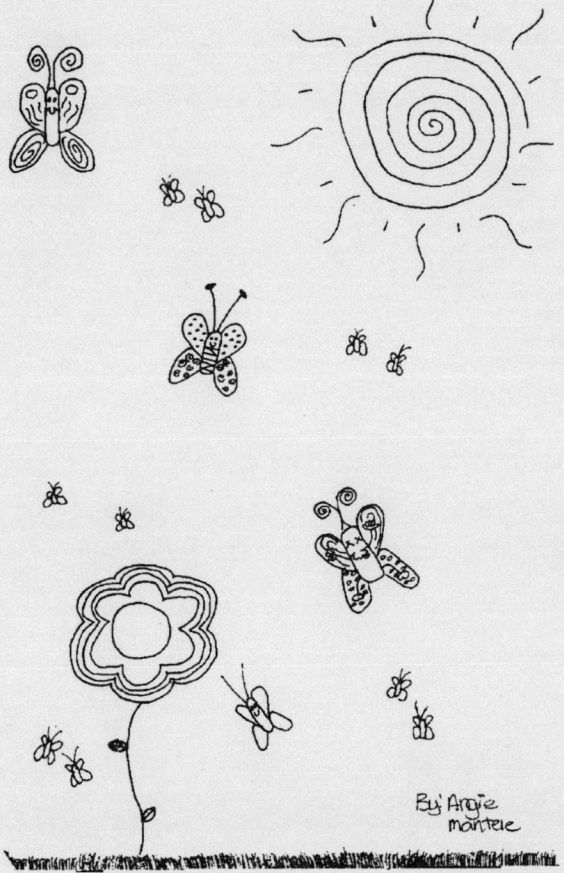

The butterfly is a beautiful symbol of summer . . . the image of freedom and beauty.

JUNE

June is the sixth month of the year. We are half way through the year with June being the most interesting garden month. Spring ends and summer begins in the northern hemisphere around June 21 or 22. Trees and shrubs are at their peak of freshness. More flowers bloom in the month of June than at any other time of the year. June is especially noted for the blooming of roses. The blossoms on the fruit trees have had their appearance and small fruit is just about to appear. Bees move from flower to flower gathering nectar. The saying of a bee keeper is "A swarm of bees in June is worth a silver spoon". As bird watchers we will notice the parent birds bringing the baby birds their food. The martins have all arrived, their melodious song is like music to my ears. Already the sparrows and starlings are sneaking their nests into empty compartments. As martin colony owners, we continue to remove these nests every week to help the martins have a home. Dusting each compartment with diatomacoeus earth is very important. Even if there are only eggs in the nest, this is one step ahead of the tiny mites those nasty sparrows and starlings bring with them. The starling will poke his long beak into the martin nest and break the eggs. Each egg broken is one less martin. The martins come from Brazil to our northern hemisphere just to raise their fledglings. This is why it is so important to help them along.

June has special days to celebrate. The earliest if Flag Day. The United States celebrates this day on June 14. We should be proud of our flag adopted by Congress in 1777.

Then we celebrate Fathers Day on the third Sunday of the month. Honoring our fathers has been the center of family activities since the beginning of time. Is it any wonder why June is believed to be the most popular month for weddings. The gem for June is the pearl. It is one of the most valuable gems. Pearls differ from other gems. Most gems are minerals mined beneath the earth. Pearls are formed inside the shells of oysters, taking several years for the particle to be completely formed.

The June bugs are usually seen at night when light attracts them. June bugs eat the young leaves of trees and shrubs, often causing a lot of damage. They deposit their eggs in the ground in meadows and grassy regions. Their larvae of white grubs with brown heads burrow into the soil in autumn and stay there two years or more. The natural control is milky spore.

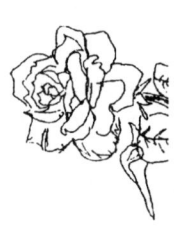

The rose has become the symbol of fragrance and beauty. The hybrid teas are ever blooming, floribundas, climbing rose and shrub rose, all growing in many different kinds of soil which thrive well under cultivation. The best location is a plot protected from cold winds, open to sunlight several hours of a day. A well drained, rich loam is usually the best soil for roses. The rose family is one of the most important of the plant kingdom. Fruit trees such as apple, pear or cherry are only a few of the rose family. Ornamental trees such as Mountain Ash and Hawthorn also belong to the rose family. There is nothing I enjoy more than to walk through my garden in this month of June with the sweet aroma of the Mountain Ash trees, Russian Olive shrubs, and flowers all in bloom. We should consider reading and learning about the trees in our own yards. I did a study of the benefits of common trees grown in most back yards.

TREES: THEIR VALUE AND WHY WE NEED TO ENCOURAGE ANNUAL PLANTING:

The benefits we receive from growing trees are many. <u>They expel their weight in Nitrogen every day and they immobilize Carbon Dioxide</u>. Tree roots tap subsoil minerals through the leaves. Leaves fall to decay and nourish soil surface. Different patterns of leaves make different sounds as the winds pick up a frequency for a musical sound for specific birds. This is how the birds pick their partner in mating and in picking their tree to build a nest. The wood of the willow family is of little use except for charcoal. Poplars and Cottonwoods are rapid growth with scaly and unusual resin coated buds. This sticky resin is gathered by honey bees for sealing crevices in their hives which beekeepers call Propoles. Fir, Spruce and Hemlock supply most of the tree pulpwood for paper. Just some of the materials we get from trees are edible fruits, coffee, syrup, spices, resin from the oily gum of trees and turpentine. Paper is the most important of all tree products. We should plant new trees every year. The very act of doing so is a humble offering to the earth. This planting then, is an act of prayer. As we walk on a cool, damp morning the wind gently moves across the blades of grass. I find myself suddenly conscious of the wonder and beauty of what has gone unseen just the day before. Can we not be a part of nature by planting a tree so that in ten years someone else can see this beauty of our handiwork?

LOMBARDY POPLAR: This tree was introduced into this country in colonial times and it has since been extensively planted as an ornamental tree that grows to a height of one hundred feet. It is a short lived tree, sending suckers from its dead trunk. The wood is of no value. Their tall narrow spike-like crowns are familiar to most people.

APPLE TREE: Leaves vary from long to oval to broadly ovate and short tipped. The familiar fruit sets on after an overly abundance of flowering. The apple can be sweet or sour. Wild apple trees grow everywhere from discarded cores. The wood of the apple tree is heavy, hard, tough and close grained. It's good for firewood. Some is used in cabinet making. The fruits are used by humans and also domestic animals such as cattle, deer, fox and raccoon.

SILVER MAPLE: The leaves are a bright green above and a silvery white beneath. They are deeply 5 lobed, with pointed or slightly rounded sinuses. Sometimes it is confused with the Red Maple, but it may readily be distinguished by the terminal lobes which usually have two shorter lobes and sides which slope inward. The fruits are the largest produced by any of the native maples with divergent wings 1½ to 2¼" long. They seed very easily wherever they fall. The wood is quite hard, but brittle. It's neither strong nor durable and is used for cheap furniture, pulpwood, boxes and crates. Syrups and sugar are sometimes made from the sap, but the yield is less than Sugar Maple.

RUSSIAN OLIVE: This is a hardy tree with a shaggy brown bark. The leaves are a silvery gray and they bear a very aromatic scented yellow flower in early spring. It grows fast to a height of thirty feet. It resists drought, pests and pollution. It is sometimes planted as a hedge which can be trimmed. It is economical to plant. This tree has sharp thorns.

MOUNTAIN ASH: There is no end to showy, fruit bearing Mountain Ash tree. It is also related to the rose family. It grows in cool temperature regions of the Northern hemisphere and grows wild in Europe, North America and northern Asia. In the cooler Southern Hemisphere you find them only as treasured garden specimens. Its feathery leaflets as leaves are ash like and soft to touch, with heavenly scented white flowerettes early in spring. The tiny fruits hang in large clusters for the birds to enjoy from late fall into winter.

RED MAPLE: These lobes are much less deeply lobed than the Silver Maple with a V shaped senuses and sides slop outward. Color is dark green with reddish tint. The bark is light gray with a smooth trunk. It grows seventy to eighty feet tall. The wood is moderately heavy, soft and neither strong or durable. It is used for furniture, boxes, crates and wood pulp. It is one of the first trees to blossom in spring and in autumn the foliage turns a brilliant red.

CHERRY TREE: The leaves are oblong-oval with rounded bases and rather taper pointed tips. A dull green color above with paler underneath. Fruits are red flesh, may be sweet or tart. In Europe the wood is often used for interior finishes, making furniture and musical instruments. Birds are very fond of the fruits and are instrumental in distributing the tree over the countryside.

GREEN ASH: Fast growing with winged clusters of flowers in early spring, maturing in autumn. Seeds are food for woodducks, quail, cardinals, finches and squirrels. The light brown wood is hard and strong and is used for tool handles, oars, paddles, baseball bats, tennis rackets and frames. Green Ash is widely planted for shade.

BLACK WALNUT: A native of Persia and believed to have been brought from Europe with the returning armies of Alexander the Great. It is still the best species, both for nuts and beautiful grained lumber. Grows slowly, bearing fragrant compound leaves with up to 13 leaflets and flowers in small greenish catkins. The oval pointed nut ripens in a greenish husk which sloughs away. The hulls were used as a dye in pioneer days. A fine crop of young plants grow every year by a forgetful squirrel which so busied himself all summer, burying the nuts. This tree is the most valuable and high praised timber tree. It is the queen of American cabinet woods and leading gun stock wood.

PEAR TREE: Pear trees bloom very early and a lot like apples, but have a different structure. The stalks of pear fruit are thicker than apples and do not join onto the fruit in a hollow. They are short stemmed. They grow wild in Europe, Asia and Africa, but not in America. The leaves are rounder and shinier than the apple. Pears are propagated from seed or by grafting cultivated varieties of wild pear stock. The wood is sometimes used for tool handles, knife handles and wood engraving.

FLOWERING CRAB APPLE: The original crab apple has white or pink flowers and is rather thorny. There are many species of the apple tree. The purple crab is most common in the northern hemisphere and is a decorative, small tree with bronzy leaves and flowers of deep purple. The fruits are purplish red and are used to make jelly. Apples are a member of the rose family, a fact which is not surprising if you look closely at their flowers and leaves.

LOCUST (COMMON): This tree is also known as Black, Yellow or White Locust. Usually grown on deep rich, moist soils. The wood is heavy, very hard and strong. It is used extensively for posts, railroad ties and ship building. It is subject to trunk damage by the locust borer and leaf damage by the leaf miner which causes premature browning and death of foliage. In May drooping clusters of pea-like, fragrant blossoms are quite attractive.

A tree expelling its weight in nitrogen each day is only one of the benefits of a tree. Other benefits are the filtering of the air, use of wood, shade it provides, homes for birds and falling leaves to decay into humus which helps replenish the roots in the coming year.

The first fruits of the season are ready to be picked. Our family's favorite time of the year is the first fresh ripe strawberry. Growing strawberries in narrow rows with a thick layer of mulch between the rows makes it easier to pick them. Removing the stem and freezing quickly on cookie sheets enables you to package the berries in containers the same day. This way of freezing allows you to take out what you need in later use throughout the year. A fresh strawberry glazed pie is a treat for a meal at home or a pot luck. Jams prepared from fresh strawberries can be a great gift to a shut in or the new family just moved into the neighborhood. Freeze some jams for later use. The strawberries are not through bearing and the first glimpse of red raspberries are showing up. Yes indeed, it is now a busy everyday chore of something needing to be done in the garden. These fruits are a good cash crop. Word of mouth and a good product is your best selling tool. As I pick the red raspberries from the strong canes that had been pruned back last fall, it is easy to work through the patch, being very careful not to damage the fruiting canes. Raspberries are a fast, perishable fruit, so care must be taken to keep them cool until sold. I have the Heritage variety which is an everbearer. These plants were set out in a one foot wide row by the good priest, Father Louis White, and myself. Five feet away from the row Father White suggested planting a row of Poplar trees on the east side. He said that these trees would have a dual purpose...grow fast and give shade while I pick the berries, and their leaves would blow between the canes for a natural mulch. It was a very good arrangement. Heritage bear heavily either in spring (June), or fall (October) in my Zone 4. One thing for sure, you do get a crop every year.

The garden is growing very fast this month. The green, bronze and ruby lettuces are the beauties of the salad bowl. The early planted radishes, peas and green beans are plentiful, along with setting heads of small Golden Acre cabbages. The tiller used in preparing your seed beds should have no use for at least three months. A stirring of the soil with a hoe or tined instrument should be the only physical work done with the soil. I still am a firm believer in a foliar feeding. This can be done at any time up to the blossom stage of fruit or vegetable. I never spray my lettuce because they are pretty much insect free and the cool nights and sunny days make them grow very well. Using the fish emulsion and sea weed foliar feeding on the tomatoes is essential at this time. It makes the plant stems stronger and adds nitrogen to the leaves. Remember to do your foliar misting in late evening or very early morning as this is the time the pores of the plant are open to accept the nutrients. Potato plants are growing fast. A misting of foliar feeding is needed to ward off the potato beetle and/or aphids. You receive benefits from foliar misting. What falls off the plant feeds the soil, especially if a mulch is used to absorb every droplet. Mulch also has a dual purpose. It keeps the soil moist, cool and weed free. Then as it decomposes it feeds the soil so the soil can feed the plant as it grows. Nature is so silent as it helps mankind that often we cannot see with our ordinary eye how it works with us.

If we are observing our gardens, orchards and lawns, we will see the beneficial insects at work. If we study nature we will learn every destructive insect has a predator. This is what we call balance. This is when a camera is beneficial for our research during our leisure hours.

The growing herbs are almost ready to set their first flowers. This is the time to cut them, selecting what you will want to dry. Common herbs like parsley, which is called "King of the Herbs", can be snipped all summer long. It has many uses, such as in stews, soups, garnishes or juices. Parsley is high in Vitamin A, C, iron and calcium.

The borage, thyme, basils and mints are all ready to cut for drying. A real good rule to follow is to plant a new herb and new vegetable each year. This broadens your menu and also your desire to learn about different plants.

As you walk through your garden you should be observing the earthworm castings. Earthworms will not survive in dry, water logged, sandy, salty, acidic soil or soil low in organic matter or calcium. They live in vertical burrows and make their way through soil by pushing aside looser soil. Earthworms eat dead organic matter that is in the soil or dead leaves and mulch that lies on top. They digest plant matter and after using their food, excrete what remains as castings on the surface of the soil. This helps to improve the soil by speeding decomposition of organic matter. it increases fertility and corrects P.H., all of which helps to improve your crop. The more you encourage earthworms, the more valuable your land will be.

The tiny trichogramma wasp is best know of all egg parasites. It attacks over 200 species of pest insects and has been used successfully against most moth and butterfly eggs. The trichogramma wasp lays its eggs in the eggs of the host pests. In due time the trichogramma eggs hatch into larva which feed on the immature pest while inside the host egg. Trico larva complete its development inside pest eggs and emerges as an adult. Then the cycle begins again. Fifteen thousand tricogramma are sufficient for a moderate sized garden. Three releases two weeks apart as soon as leaves are fully emerged. The trico wasp measure1/32" and deposits 25 eggs in one host. Life cycle from egg to adult wasp is 10 days.

The trichogramma primarily attacks worms such as cotton bollworm, corn earworm, corn looper, Oriental fruit moth, imported cabbage worm and tomato horn worm.

Each vegetable planted should be ready to use. It's a great value to be able to pick a different vegetable each day for our meals. Sugar Snap peas, green beans, tiny sweet carrots, red ruby beets, champion radish and many of the lettuce family should be at their peak. Be sure to incorporate a plan to build a compost pile from all residues of the vegetable leaves, plus your discarded weeds, layering as you go. A little soil, manure, and old straw or hay residue are all good sources to

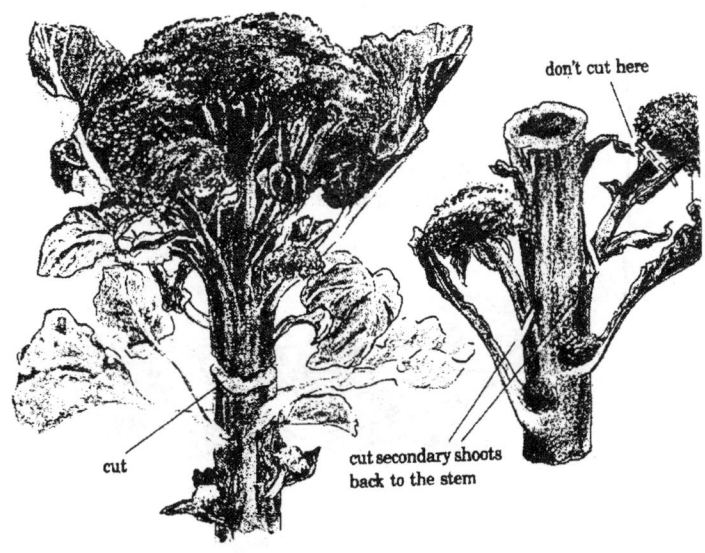

work with.

These next two months are the most appropriate months to make a completed compost. Use the solar sun to help heat the pile, always remembering to use an aerobic bio-dynamic compost starter that has the beneficial micro-organisms to help decompose the pile of residue. More details on composting will be in the next two months' reports.

A great garden month gone by!

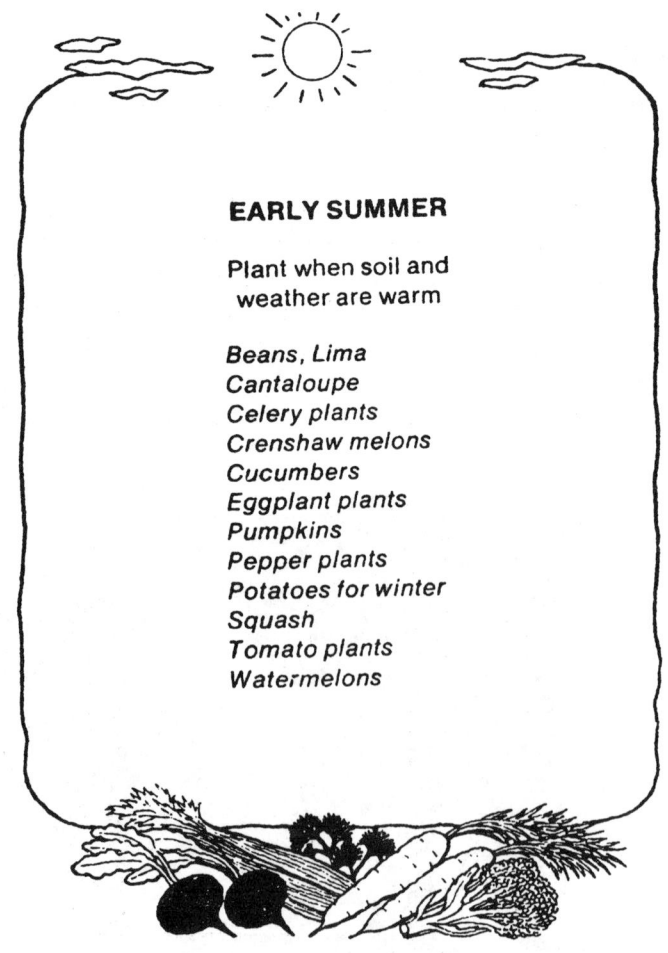

EARLY SUMMER

Plant when soil and weather are warm

Beans, Lima
Cantaloupe
Celery plants
Crenshaw melons
Cucumbers
Eggplant plants
Pumpkins
Pepper plants
Potatoes for winter
Squash
Tomato plants
Watermelons

JULY

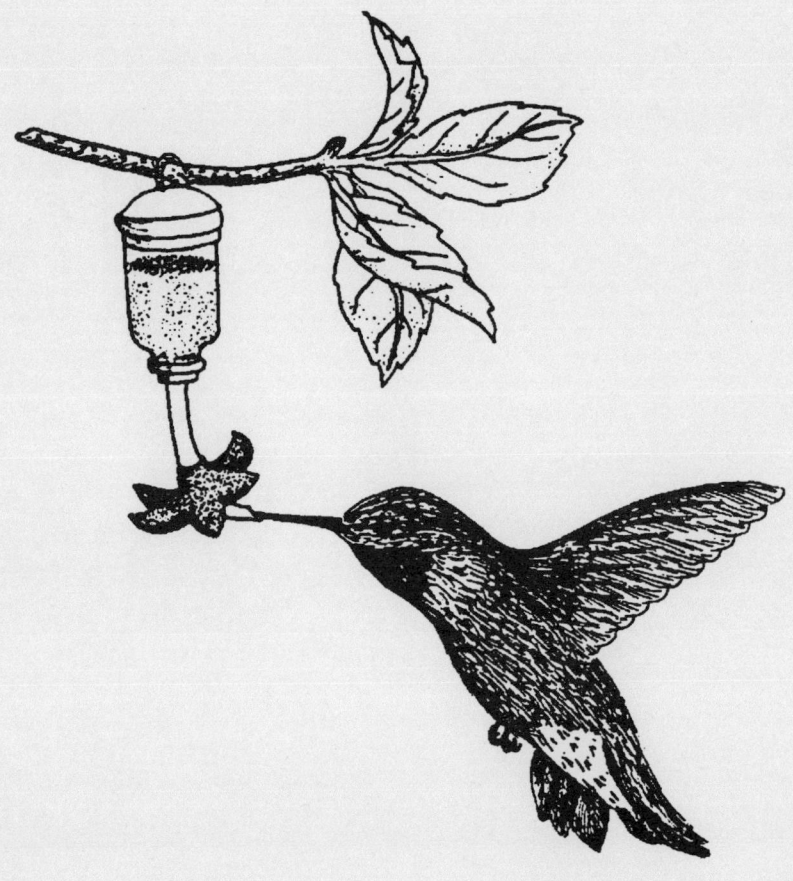

They're bold.
They are brilliant.
They are beneficial.
The humming bird is a joy to watch as
they hover at my nectar feeder.

JULY

Beauty repeats itself. Just turning a page on the calendar does not mean the beauty of the June garden is gone. July spills over many true beauties of its own. Year after year the perennial flowers pour out arrays of color. The daisy, snapdragons, phlox and coreopsis are all in their glory, nestled in by annuals of poppy, cosmos, bachelor buttons, zinnias and marigolds. As we see a barren spot we tuck in an extra plant for added color. A daily walk through the garden is necessary to keep checking to see if weeds are popping up. This month we encounter dry spells so care must be taken to mulch where possible, especially if watering is necessary. Mulch holds moisture, plus keeps the soil cool. The potatoes and tomatoes should be mulched now. Nitrogen is now needed and a bath of fish emulsion of three tablespoons to one gallon of water is a good insurance policy. The mulch will be benefited by what drips off the plant.

Cucumbers are prolific by now. Hopefully the cucumber beetle has not visited your patch. There are many suggestions of how to keep them away. I believe a combination of many practices help, but soil balance is the key. A strong plant is necessary too. I've used a soap solution, "Heavens Green", the past two years with the best results yet. This product contains beneficial herbs that I feel are very helpful.

We have more fruits and vegetables to pick, can, freeze, dry or sell. Cherries are ready to pick. This is a chore about once every 10 days. I like to juice mine, freeze the juice and then bag the pulp to freeze for pies, cobblers or cherry bars.

The zucchini are ready. Seems like every gardener plants too much squash. It's so hard not to plant the entire package, hoping at least a few plants will survive the squash borer or squash bugs and beetles. You need to keep a constant watch over the patch. To beat the borer you must spot the adults working the vines in midday. The first sign is a sawdust-like mass that shows up where the larvae enters the stem. The simplest solution is to inject a B.T. preparation using a syringe above the point of entry. Another solution is to cut with a sharp knife, slitting the stem, finding the borers, removing them and then healing the wound by covering it with mounded moist soil. This heals shut rather quickly. The squash bug is another pesty problem. These mature very rapidly and do a lot of damage quickly. Spraying with pyrethrum or Heavens Green insecticide soap is a help. Cutting off the leaf bearing clusters of eggs is a step ahead of the adult bugs. One needs to be alert to stay ahead of this problem. The insect parasite Tachinid fly can destroy up to ninety percent of the squash bugs in an area. These flies lay their eggs on the squash bugs, then the fly larva bores into the body of the bug. Attract these adult flies by planting dill, parsley, fennel, buckwheat or amarenth.

Just because this seems to be the hottest month of gardening with a good variety of vegetables ready to eat, can, dry or sell does not mean we are through planting or planning. This is the month we must start to seed our fall crops. The cold crops do much better in late fall when you are free of most of the insects that bother in the summer. Plant radish seed every three weeks to have a supply of tender radishes. Seed between rows of mulch where the soil already is cooler and moist. Plant head lettuce, beets, spinach and kohlrabi and set out small plants of cauliflower and broccoli which grew from the spring seeding.

Renew the mulch around the roses and perennials to encourage longer flowering. Green peppers love a cool soil. These plants are fully grown and need a layer of mulch to prevent the fruit from aborting. Always plant peppers in an area that's partly shaded in the afternoon. Peppers do not do well in ninety degree heat.

Let us not forget to feed our compost pile. Any residue from lawn, garden or kitchen scraps, other than meats, are most welcome to build your pile to a good sized heap. This is what helps to build heat for decomposition. Add some water if needed to keep a moist structure of thirty percent.

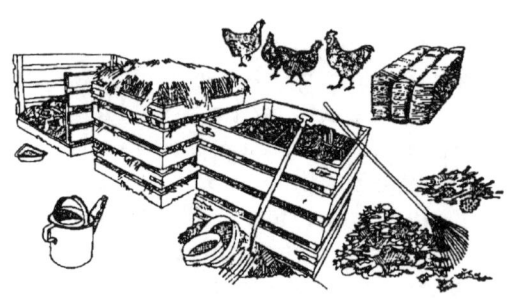

Picnic time is a sure way to celebrate in this seventh month of the year. The celebration of Independence Day is an early start and one we all remember, even as little children. When I was growing up I remember the fourth of July for different reasons. It was indeed hay making weather. Our hay was hauled in on a wagon loosely stacked and driven by a team of tame horses. A wooden ladder was built in front for the driver of this team to stand by. My father would neatly layer the hay as the hay loader would bring the hay onto the wagon. His idea of a good packed load of hay was piled high, even over my head as I stood on this wooden ladder. One soon learned to pull your collar tight so the chaff wouldn't get down your neck. That was only half of the work. Load by load we would drive to the barn with a huge open door near the roof. A big hay fork driven with a pulley in the peak of the barn would drop down onto this load of hay. One person would stick the prongs of the fork into the hay. Another person on the opposite side of the barn would drive a horse pulling a huge rope through this pulley in order to raise the hay to the hay loft. Then two people would spread the fork full of hay in layers in the hay loft. This was an important part of handling the loose hay because when feeding this hay next winter it had to be peeled back as it was layered and thrown down a chute to feed the cattle.

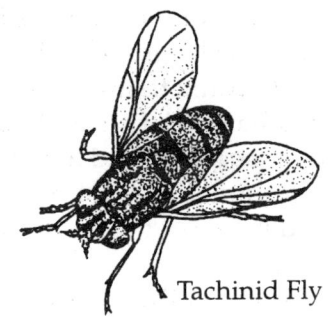
Tachinid Fly

The Fourth of July also meant berry picking time. Dad and anyone who could walk in a timber had their small bucket tied around their waist with a rope to help pick berries. We had to ask permission to pick in another farmer's timber. The pay for the berries was half of what you picked. This was a hot and uncomfortable task. What we ate in the timber was our salary. My father was very honest in bringing the filled buckets to show the owners our fruits. Maybe this is why I still like to pick my red raspberries in my garden. I'm not sure I would trample through the woods and pick berries in the nineties. One sure thing we knew when we got home mother would have a good meal ending up with berries and cream from the milk we separated ourselves by turning a hand crank on our separator. The chores in the thirties were much different than today. As each Independence day comes and goes I am thankful for the convenience of planning a family gathering picnic at a park.

The flower of the month is the Water Lily. This flower takes a special place in a pond or man made water garden with a recirculating pump. I appreciate the lilies, iris and colombine that grow and bloom heartily in my yard each July. Mosquito time is here. All one needs to do is sit in your lawn swing to be visited by this pesky insect. The mosquito spreads disease in all regions of the world. All mosquitoes begin life as eggs laid either on the surface of water or in shaded areas of trees. From eggs they turn to larvae, growing very rapidly to the pupae stage with a time frame of two weeks to become an adult. Mass spraying has been done with great side effects. This is why I love my purple martins so much. Be sure to work with the martins. They love to be talked to. Keep their homes comfortable by dusting with diatomaoues earth to protect their fledglings from the mites. Every week is not too many times to check in their nests to see the fledglings grow. This month is a good time to count the birds. The fledglings will soon fly and then you will not be able to count them. I take an inventory each year of the number of eggs, eggs hatched and fledglings that live. This way I know how many colonies I have and how many new birds to plan for next year. Yes, you may think it is a lot of work, but it's well spent when we can say our yard is free of mosquitoes.

Ruby is the gem for July. It's another rare mineral of aluminum oxide called Corundum. The finest rubies come from Burma. Garnets coming from North Carolina and Arizona are often sold under misleading names. This stone is also the symbol of the fortieth wedding anniversary.

This month is also vacation time. School is out and the youngsters can learn from travel as much as from a textbook. But don't forget to include the youngsters in your garden work. They should be given short rows to plant what they wish. The younger you start a child in the garden, the more likely he or she is to have a worthwhile hobby for the rest of his or her life. It is important to have their help in picking and preparing food for storage.

This month has so many fruits and vegetables to preserve for future meals. Let's take advantage of this great opportunity for good health by eating good food.

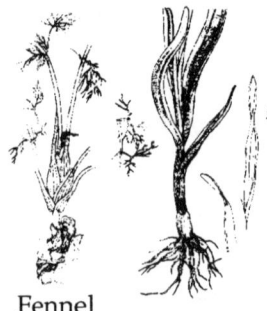
Fennel Garlic

Lawns are slowly calming down to one cutting a week. Learning to cut a little higher will save the lawns. Leave the grass clippings lie on top to serve as food for the soil.

In this hot month the radishes have a tendency to go to seed. It's a good practice to leave one row. The seeds will form and then dry in the pod, fall to the ground and be mulched by the leaves of the plant. Then when spring comes you will see a bed of radishes soon show up after the snow and frost have left the soil moist and cool. Try not to till on this spot when preparing your soil for spring work.

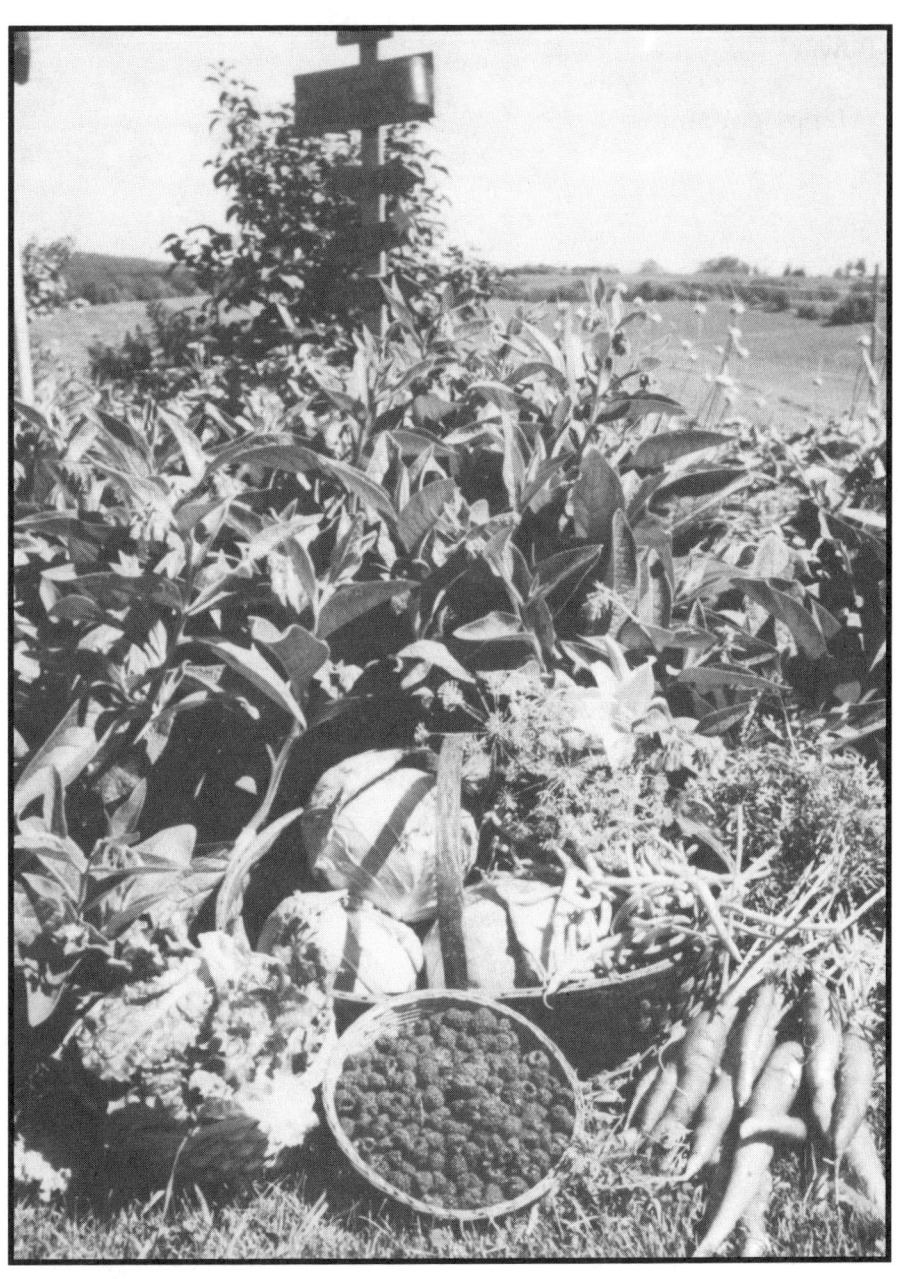

A bountiful harvest of fruit, vegetables and herbs.

A good practice I have found to be very beneficial is to visit other gardeners to exchange ideas, extra plants, a new herb or just a bouquet of flowers.

Happy gardening!

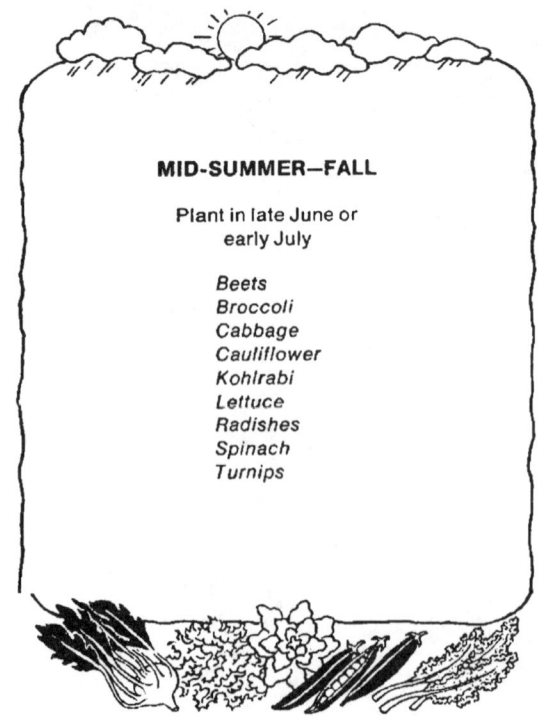

MID-SUMMER—FALL

Plant in late June or early July

Beets
Broccoli
Cabbage
Cauliflower
Kohlrabi
Lettuce
Radishes
Spinach
Turnips

AUGUST

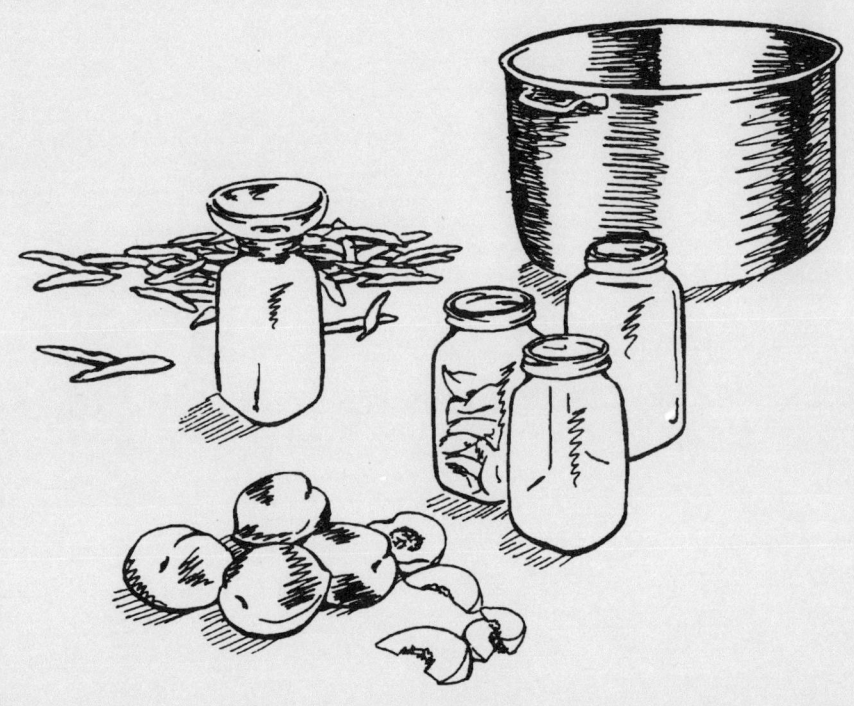

In a busy summers day
I always find a way.
To can food is an art
with my garden to help do it's part.

AUGUST

This is a serious month for getting things done. The weather is usually hot and dry. Tomatoes need to be canned, juiced or made into soups, sauces and catsup. The cabbages are bursting, wanting to be prepared into Kraut. Almost all the vegetables need attention this month. Potato vines are drying up. If the mulch is not covering the hills, digging now is necessary. Potatoes exposed to the sun turn green and are dangerous to eat. Some of the vegetables are on the decline in bearing and these make good soups. Drying these small amounts works great. The end product is easy to store and they also make nice Christmas gifts. The onion stem has bent over and started to dry. Stored properly, newer varieties of the onion keep from four to 18 months. Only the right varieties for your climate and length of days, stored under cool, dry conditions will survive this long. The sweet Spanish and Bermuda onions are more palatable and easier on your eyes to peel and slice. The problem is they sprout easily and store poorly. The longer storage onions are Yellow Globe, Spartan Sleeper or Improved Buccaneer. These are adapted to the northern climate with long maturing days. The recommended time to pull onions is when the plant tops fall over and the bulbs pull easily. If they are hard to lift out of the ground it means the root is still growing. Wait until the green top turns brown and the neck of the onion no longer feels slippery or slick. Onions are best cured in a ventilated shed. Even a fan to create moving air greatly reduces the chance of disease and rotting. During winter cool but not freezing basements make good storage sites. Other practices are braiding, storing in mesh bags or nylon pantyhose and hanging up to let the air circulate around them.

This month we should harvest our garlic, treating the bulbs just like the onion. After the cloves are dried they can be braided in nice arrangements. Planting the stray cloves is assurance of a crop the following year. Each clove must be broken apart to grow a good sized bulb the following year. Cloves should be incorporated with canning pickles and other vegetables used in soups. Any surplus can be sold at farmers markets. The excess sweet corn, cucumbers, squash, apples, pears and other excess crops should bring in the needed cash for planting in your garden.

Drying fruits and vegetables can be solar sun dried or done in an oven or dehydrator. Chili peppers hung on a string, then hung up on the south side of a shed works great. The beans and peas should ripen on the plant. They are easily podded when time and labor permit. This is a good children's project on a hot, sunny day under the shade tree in your yard. August is fair month. Your best vegetable could take a blue ribbon. How about entering your prize pie in a contest? The truth of your produce is in the eating.

Many gardeners overlook the potential of a fall garden, never even thinking of replanting in midsummer. Seeds germinate quickly, seedlings shoot up within a week, and yields are impressive, despite a late start. After harvesting spring and summer crops I apply a good source of compost. The sprouted seeds and seedlings are fed a manure tea, followed by a misting of fish emulsion of three tablespoons to one gallon of water. Leaf lettuce is directly seeded in the mulched area to hold the moisture. Kohlrabi grows fast and is so tender and sweet up to frost time. Weeds are less of a problem in fall, so five minutes of daily hoeing is all that's necessary. Gardening is a healthy hobby. The food is the best quality and the exercise is so beneficial. Sweet corn galore! Every household eats corn on the cob in season. Eat. freeze, can or dry enough for your own use, then sell the surplus. Any corn that's too mature can be left to dry in the husk, then ground for corn meal. This is much sweeter than other corn meals.

As the month ends I start to build up my soil with a cover crop. To keep the humus content high I sow wheat and sometimes rye among the still growing vegetables and flowers. It makes good growth by the end of October. It dies down in winter, but starts to grow again in spring. Sometimes I must mow the wheat or rye off as the growth gets too high. I till only enough of a patch that I will plant in one day. Therefore, some of this green cover grows to fast. This also has a twofold purpose. It is a soil builder, but also helps hold the soil in place reducing erosion.

It seems like we are bouncing from one job to another, but that is what August is all about. Not done with one task, another is waiting.

We haven't talked about the fruit in season. Pears are melting on the tree, so full of juice the honey bees are drawing the sweet juice from the overripe ones. Pears are very perishable and need attention right after picking. The apples are dropping, waiting to be used in a fresh pie or cobbler. Melons are in good supply, which makes one wonder which fruit to eat first. Juicing uses up a large amount of abundant perishable fruit. These juices can be frozen for later use.

Now the task of making compost. Hopefully, all the excess lawn trimmings, vegetable waste, kitchen garbage, leaves, old straw and any type of manure has been heaped up all year. One of the biggest mistakes a gardener makes in getting good compost is not making a big enough pile. It takes a heap of material to start the action of decomposition. A beneficial bacteria for an enhancer will make your residue decompose faster and these micro-organisms will benefit the finished product. This pile needs air in order to heat properly as we are working with an aerobic bacteria. By increasing the micro-organisms the pile continues to heat and decompose. One important factor is the moisture content of the residue. If it is not a 30% moisture it will not heat up to decompose. Mixing some soil with it sometimes helps to get the bacterial action going. Layered properly I find it is not necessary to add soil. When completed it produces a dark rich material any good gardener would recognize as valuable as gold. Composting is not new. As a child I remember pitching out the gutter manure during the winter months with a pitch fork. Then in the spring before planting we had to use a shovel to pick up this same manure, turned into compost by itself. Our soil, plants and animals then had the good, beneficial bacteria in them. Today chemical fertilizer has killed all the beneficial life in the soil. This is why the roots of our cornstalks will not rot away on their own. Today landfills will not accept compostable refuse so the law forces the homeowner to compost. It's the best fertilizer a gardener can use. don't cut yourself short by not having your own compost pile.

Golden Rod, asters, fall mums and many annual flowers brighten the landscape. The insects are noisier and more numerous than in any other month. Some birds are already preparing to fly south. All the fledglings of the purple martins can now fly, so by the 15th of August they have sung their good-byes. We can tell a day or two before they leave. All of the birds are flying around like crazy, taking their last mosquitoes with them. Then they sit on the power lines as if they are all lining up to take off together. Yes, it's a sad day because now the bug problem must be handled by ourselves. It could be a week and then another group may sleep overnight, but be gone the next day. These martins are never as friendly, but doesn't it seem strange how they find their way to Brazil and back without a road map? Yes, God's creatures are great.

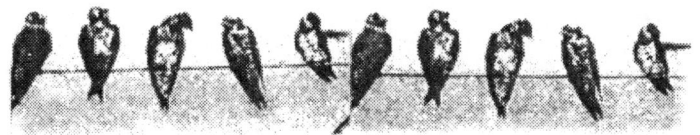

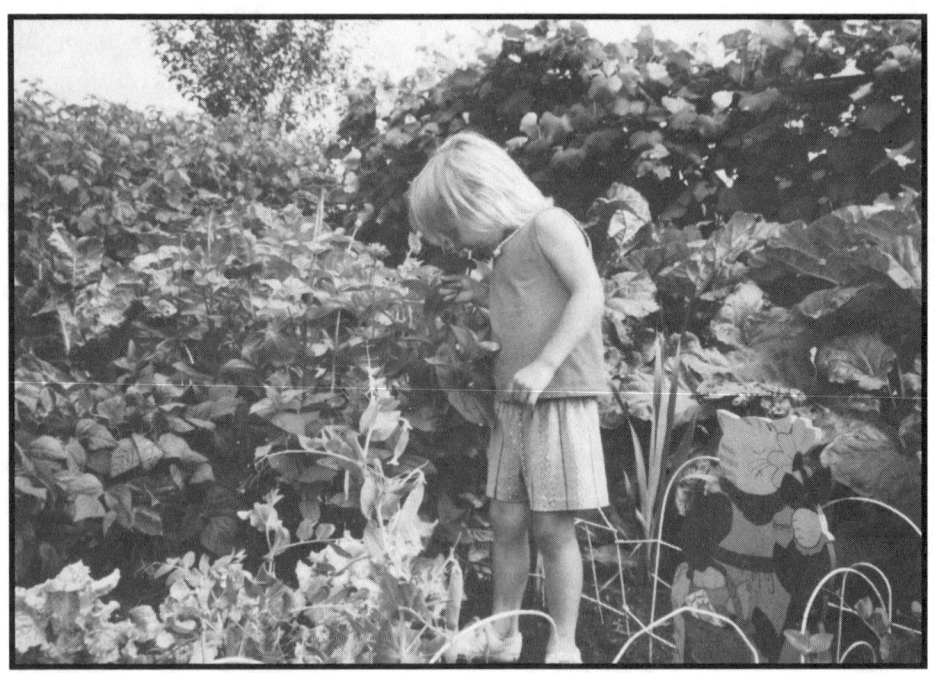
Brooke, my granddaughter taking time to smell the flowers in her own garden.

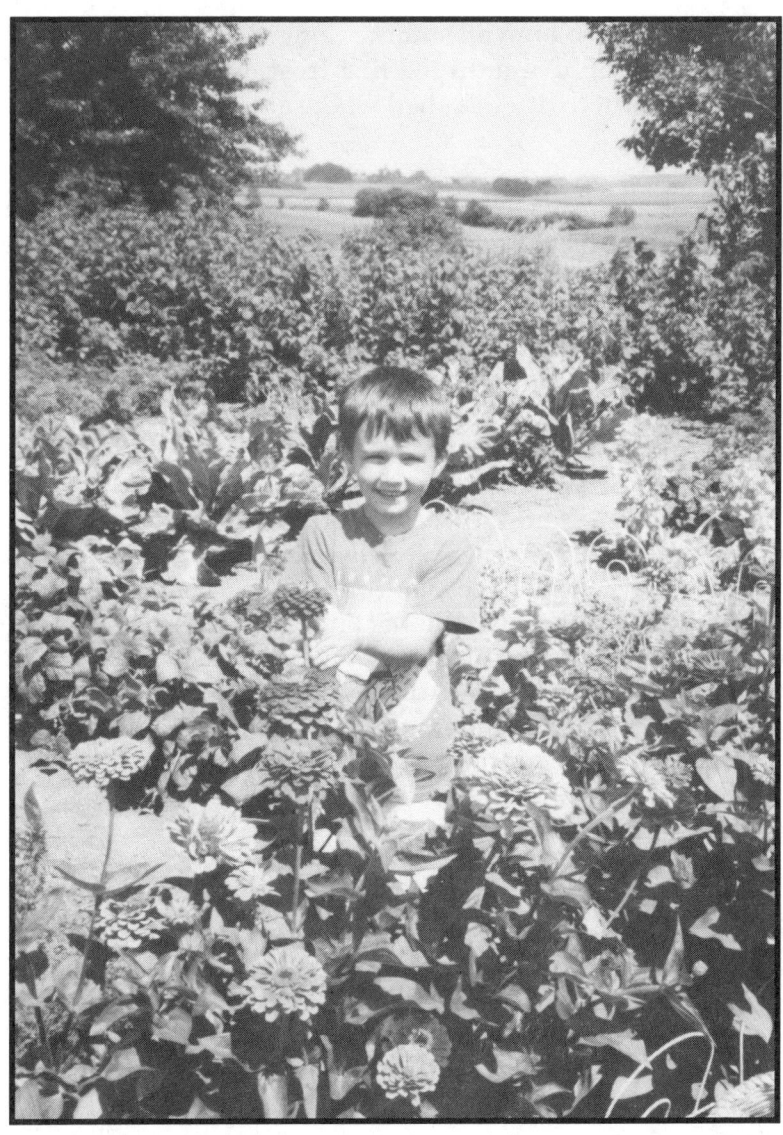
Seth, my grandson is a big help harvesting vegetables grown in his garden.

The flowers of August can be the poppies and the gladiolus. Both of these grow in abundance in many climates. The gladiola especially is a flower to enter at fairs or in flower shows. Grown from a bulb, planted early in the spring and then spacing the plantings every two weeks will guarantee flowers to bloom all summer long. When the flower dies off the green blades will live until the first frost, which is time to dig the bulbs. Lay them out to dry in a shed where air circulates. Store in a dry place over winter.

The gem of August is the sardonyx. This gem is a form of a quartz used in rings or jewelry. Jewelers can cut many sizes, shapes and designs to bring out its full color of brown, golden or blood red. Cameos are made from this gem which is found in Brazil, India, Scotland and Ireland.

The last days of August can be spent by walking through your garden, collecting seed pods from your favorite annual flowers. Harvesting potatoes, bulb onions and dried beans and preparing them for storage is the benefit reaped from the year's work. Now too, a note should be added to your garden inventory of which variety vegetable you want to plant next year. Hardy flowers like pansies, Sweet Williams and snapdragons can be planted now. Weed the strawberry bed and transplant robust new runners. Add compost to the plot, soaking the roots with a fish emulsion solution. This should guarantee the roots to set soon. Turn your compost pile again. Start a new site for more garden refuse. Never add to the pile already decomposing.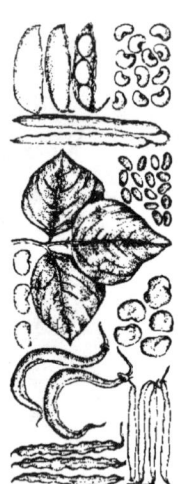

This decomposed pile will be ready to use. Always pile residue on the bare ground. This gives air and moisture from the bottom of the pile. Alternating with different types of residue will also let air build up into the pile. Shredded material will decompose more rapidly but must be turned to prevent matting down. Signs of gray material on the top or sides indicates too much heat and your residue will turn to an ash which is not beneficial to your compost. Aeriate by turning with a machine or fork. You want the best product after putting the hard work into a compost heap.

SEPTEMBER

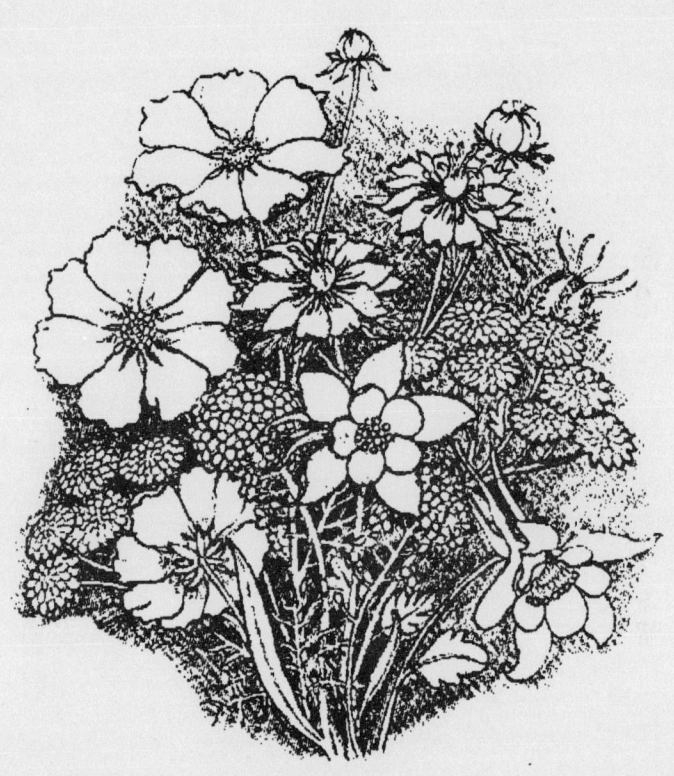

With all the autumn blaze of Golden Rod we see everywhere the Purple Aster nod. The annuals all so brightly bloom a perfect bouquet for any room.

SEPTEMBER

A view from your window to the garden on a dewy September morning requires a serious task of filming your garden. Its rewards are many. Its bountiful beauty nourishes body and soul. At this time of the year when all vegetables are in their full glory we should take the time to take an inventory on the seeds we selected and planted. Which variety did the best? Which variety was wilt resistant? Which produced more and withstood the weather extremes? In my garden the Black-seeded Simpon lettuce or Bibb and Ithaca head lettuce is hard to beat. I have learned the Thumbelina globe sized carrot is not going to be a favorite for any gardener. We can tell which variety of sweet corn produced early and is the sweetest. The cucumbers are at their peak. Ramble through your cookbooks to find new and different ways to preserve them. Farmers markets are all open and the extra surplus can be carefully picked and displayed in neat baskets, boxes or buckets. Taking orders from shut-ins or senior citizens who cannot come to the farmers market is a way of helping sell your products.

This overall inventory now needs to be written down. When the seed catalogs come one tends to forget which variety did the best. Weeding seems to be a chore every month. The secret is not to allow the weeds to go to seed. Pulled and put on a compost pile is the best way to treat them. The saying is "weeds tell you what is missing in your soil". Dandelions tell me the soil is lacking calcium. A high calcium lime is needed to correct this. At this time my most frequently asked question is, what can I do for the tomato wilt? Sorry to say, this needs to be attended to before the wilt. Mulching sure helps, but it's not the complete answer. Lack of nitrogen is a main reason for wilting of the bottom leaves. I have found that if you gave your tomato plants their bath of fish emulsion (three tablespoons to one gallon of water) all summer every 10 to 14 days you shouldn't have a real problem. By this time the plant has used up a lot of soil nutrients so I mix sea kelp in with the fish emulsion (again, three tablespoons of sea kelp and three tablespoons of fish emulsion in one gallon of water). Mist on plants after 6:00 p.m. or before 8:00 a.m. because this is the only time the pores of the plant leaf are open to accept the nutrients. If your water is chlorinated you must let it set 24 hours in the sun to draw out the chlorination. This is real important. Saving rain water would be a good practice. Maybe we need to bring out the old fashioned rain barrel.

Crickets seem to be a problem for many gardeners when tomatoes are almost ripe. A dusting of diatomaceous earth over the plants and onto the mulch will calm them down. This is a natural powder which consists of the skeletal remains of Diatom, a one cell plant-like algae. The skeleton of the Diatom contains a multitude of pores causing it to have a sponge-like structure so that good quality diatomaceous earth can absorb up to three and four times its mass of liquid water. It has 14 known trace minerals so it is a nutrient and a plant dust. It controls ants, young leaf rollers, mites, thrips and certain aphids. It can be fed to pets and animals to control ticks and fleas and can be put in their bedding and dusted in their hair. I put a handful in each chicken nest and use it on the bedding in corners and places where flies breed. It can also be used in grain storage. As a lawn insecticide, diatomaceous earth is a potent deterrent to grubs, cinch bugs, cutworms and other soil insects. Apply the dust four times a year at a rate of 25 pounds per 1500 square feet. Be sure you are using the diatomaceous earth that is milled until almost completely amorphous, which means it has no crystal-line form left to cause damage to larger organisms. Instead, it has small sharp edges which can damage tiny parasites, larvae on stored grain, in animal manure, on infected plants, and in the stomachs of livestock. Do not use the filter diatomaceous earth used for swimming pools in any type of agricultural practice.

The cucumber beetle is another pesty insect. Many things have been tried, like planting radish seed in the hill at planting time, a handful of wood ashes around the newly emerged plants, marigold interplanting, row covers or hand picking the insect, whirling them in a blender and spraying back on the plants. I am not sure if any one or combination will work. I do know the weather plays a part. Imbalance in the soil may be a reason or tolerant seed source could be the culprit. So each gardener may find help from different sources.

My best results were in 1992, when I misted the plants with an insecticidial soap I make myself. I remember when I was a little girl and my mother did not have electricity, running water or a basement. We had a wash house, heated the water in an iron kettle, had a kerosene driven wash machine and she made her own lewis lye soap. One of my chores was to take the wash water to the garden. Well, I still make the lewis lye soap, so with that and some herbs in an oil base, I make this mist. It works great on the soil itself to open it up and absorb more of the rain so that the top six to eight inches are like a sponge. I really do not know if my mother knew why she was putting the wash water on the garden, other than watering it. You see, we saved our precious water for it had to be pumped with a windmill and carried in buckets wherever we needed it.

Our onions are ready to dig when the stem has bent over and dried.

Digging carefully so as not to bruise the bulb is very important. Lay them out to dry out of the sun and rain. Or they can be braided by the stem and hung up in an outside building. Sorting and selling the nicer bulbs is a good way to reimburse you for the plants you bought in the spring. Onions contain sulfur which has already been proven to inhibit certain types of cancer. The small single multiplier onion we planted in April and May now has six bulblets to dig and dry for next year's planting. These keep very well in a basement until next planting season. The garlic can be dug very early in September. Thinking ahead for the next garden season we should be breaking these shallots apart and planting them in a bed so their growth will be well started before frost.

The dried beans are also ready to harvest, adzuki, navy, lima...all favorites of mine. I keep seeds every year to replant. A handful of the cooked variety mixed in a lettuce salad is a treat in winter time.

Now the strawberry bed has sprawled all out of shape. You can see the new tender plants along the edges. With a mower, design your row for next year, cutting away the old bed. In a day or two the leaves and stems will be dried enough to rake off and add to your compost pile. If you don't rake them off they will plug up your tiller blades. Now you can rototill this old patch out and keep the new row as wide as you like. My preference is to pick down one side, then the opposite side. Your nicest berries are on the edges. You may want to rototill this every four days until no growth is left. Then a layer of mulch of hay or straw, or cornstalk all shredded is a real life saver for weed control. It does more than control weeds. We are conserving moisture, feeding humus to the soil through decomposition and giving the beneficial micro-organisms a place to live and manufacture food for the earth worm. By taking care of a strawberry bed this way you can "walk" your bed the entire length of your garden without setting out a new bed. Being a member of the Iowa Natural Food Associates Chapter, I advertise in our quarterly newsletter for anyone wanting plants to start a new bed. Members come and dig them up, a way of sharing with others. After all, Father Louis White brought the plants to me to get a bed started. Fruit is a sure seller, with orders galore. It's time consuming and they are perishable. Again, word of mouth is your best advertising.

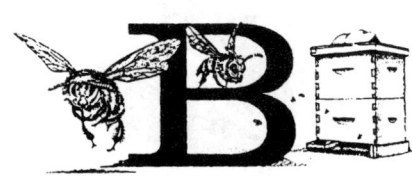

It is still the allergy season with the pollen count very high. My experience to get rid of pollen allergies absolutely has been to eat sunflower seeds with comb honey. The wax from the comb contains a natural penicillin and both should be chewed together. The honeycomb can be taken from the hive this month. The honey bees on our farm are in a protected area near a spring and there are many trees with pollen, including apple trees, that the bees pollinate.

The fall raspberries are starting to bear now and they have a "too good to be true" flavor. Many varieties can be planted to stretch your raspberry season. Heritage is the variety I have and the only one. This patch of thirty years has never failed to bear...sometimes two large crops, always one large crop. I guess I like them because I know their pattern of growth. Their bearing time fits in perfect with my garden chores. They bear in late June and early July when not a lot of canning is being done. Then they bear again in late September and early October when my canning is slowing down. I just love them the way they are. Most of my crop is sold, now that my family has left to raise their own families. Those that I freeze I spread out on a cookie sheet which allows you to thaw only as many as you need for one meal.

Watermelon and muskmelons are at their peak right now. It gets to be a problem of what shall I eat first. Juiced and served with a mint leaf, these make delicious cool drinks on a hot summer day.

Why not have a garden tour or a potluck dinner, going from garden to garden? Every time I visit someone else's garden I learn of a short cut or new method of doing things. It's a way of self educating, sharing your experiences, successes and failures. Not every gardener grows the same thing. Father White always used to say to me, "Rita, you must grow one new vegetable every year. Discard some, but keep adding". I found that some of the new ones became our favorite vegetables. Some of these were sugar snap peas, lima bean, eggplant, adzuki bean, and this year, the parsnips. You also learn new tricks to control predators and insects. I now hang empty milk jugs in all my trees to catch the moths by saving all vinegar sauces from pickles and beets I use during the winter. Save some apple cider to turn into vinegar and use these liquids in the milk jugs. Keep the caps on, cut a circle out and hang them by the handle with a nylon. You may have to dump out 3" of moths at least three times a year and refill them with vinegar-honey liquid.

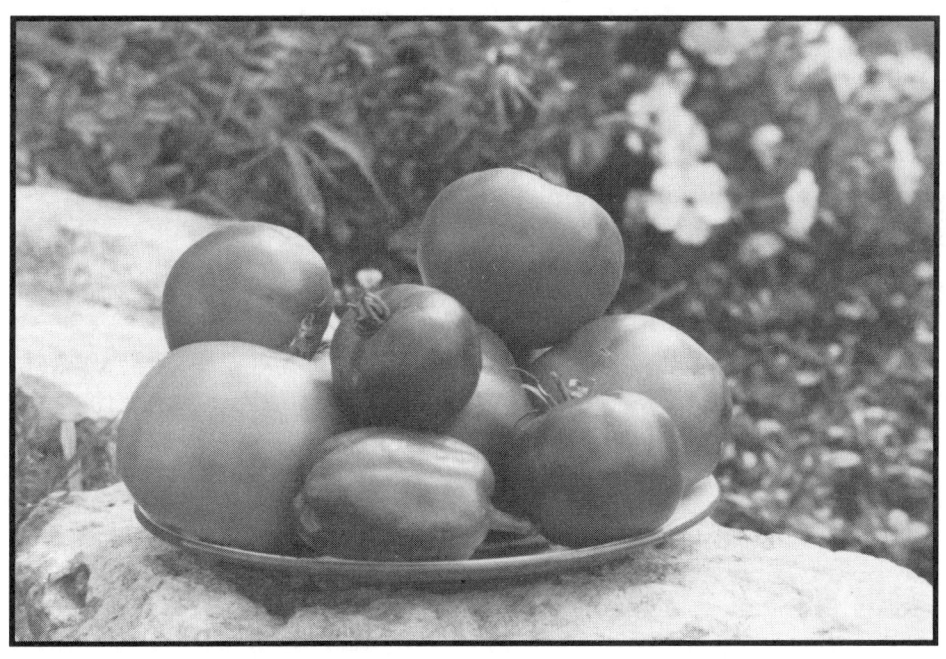
Bright red and green vegetables to add color and flavor to your meals.

Moles are bad at this time of the year. Grub is their main food and they love the mulch and lawns. Putting two or three tablespoons of Diatomaceous Earth in the runway eliminates them from using that same tunnel. Slugs can be trapped in shallow tins dug even with the ground. Stale beer, sugar water or spoiled, fermented fruit in water are good traps. Each gardener seems to have a specialty of his own and that's what sharing your garden and self educating is all about.

A garden fest is a celebration of organic gardening...a day long event where you learn from seeing, exchanging plants, bulbs, produce, and buying, selling or trading with everyone else. All you need to bring is a covered dish from a recipe you want to share and a good appetite.

Wreaths made from herbs can be hung in your kitchen and you can snitch a herb or two while cooking. Garlic braids with dried flowers are very unique. Walk timberland and pick Queen Anne's Lace, milkweed pods, daises and other interesting weeds, flowers or seed pods. Usually you can attend classes on making the wreaths or decorations, but also use your own imagination. So many crafts can be made from plants.

You are reminded of the balance of nature by just observing what is going on under your feet as you walk and note the soft feel of the soil, the decomposition of last year's leaves and the wildlife digging the soil for grubs and insect eggs.

If this job was not done in August, it is time to dig potatoes because the potato vines are all dried off. Some of the potatoes are heaving through the soil, which tells us they are done growing. It's time to dig them up and dry for winter storage. Potatoes like a soil leaning to an acid ph. scale. As soon as the potatoes are dug, work up the soil and seed wheat, rye or soybeans which are all an excellent soil cleansing crop for next season. Dry the tubers in a dark place for several days to cure them. Then store them in a cool place at forty degrees, which is an ideal temperature range for potatoes. A fifty foot garden row can yield up to one bushel. For many people, potatoes are the staple food. Potatoes are nutritious and not at all fattening. It's what you add to them that adds inches.

Picking tomatoes by the pound, peck or bushel seems to be the rule of thumb. With the interest in eating locally grown foods without chemicals, it is becoming a trend to can, freeze, preserve and juice tomatoes. A bushel weighs sixty pounds. You'll have more orders than an average gardener can supply. It is important to have uniform size when selling. Cracked, stem rot, insect damaged or not quite ripe are

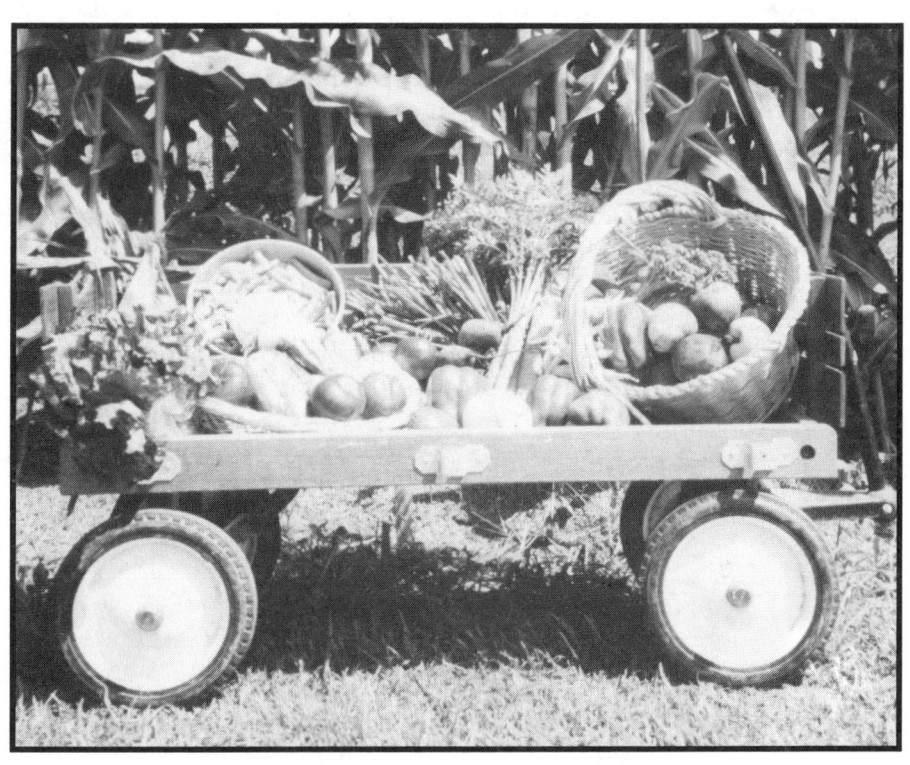

A wagon load of garden produce ready for farmers market.

not good sellers. Mulch protects rotting and insures a clean fruit. Tomato horn worms can strip your patch in a few days if left unattended. They can be hand picked in most gardens. There are two kinds...the green tomato horn worm and the brown tobacco horn worm. Caution should be taken not to destroy the horn worm with white cocoons on their backs. This is a beneficial braconids wasp egg which is very helpful to the farmer. If these eggs are seen on the horn worm, just let them be. That horn worm can do no more damage and the braconids wasp will mature to a reddish like dragonfly related to the Ichneumon fly. Both the braconids and Ichneumon control major pests. Always pick the wilted leaves and destroy them so they do not harbor disease. Keeping tomatoes in cages prevents rotting, but I feel it slows the ripening because the sun cannot reach through heavy foliage. Mulching only after blossoming starts as the plant likes hot sun on the soil up to this stage. Then when mulched the plant now needs a cool soil to mature. Slow growth and yellow leaves tell me the plant is starving for nitrogen. A daily walk through the garden keeps you in tune with their daily needs. You can control your ripening by picking the tomatoes and putting them in a sunny place. This will assure you of a nice amount to can or sell. The tomatoes you take to the farmers market must be uniform in size and ripening.

Good luck and turn a new leaf on your calendar.

FRAGRANT FLOWERS

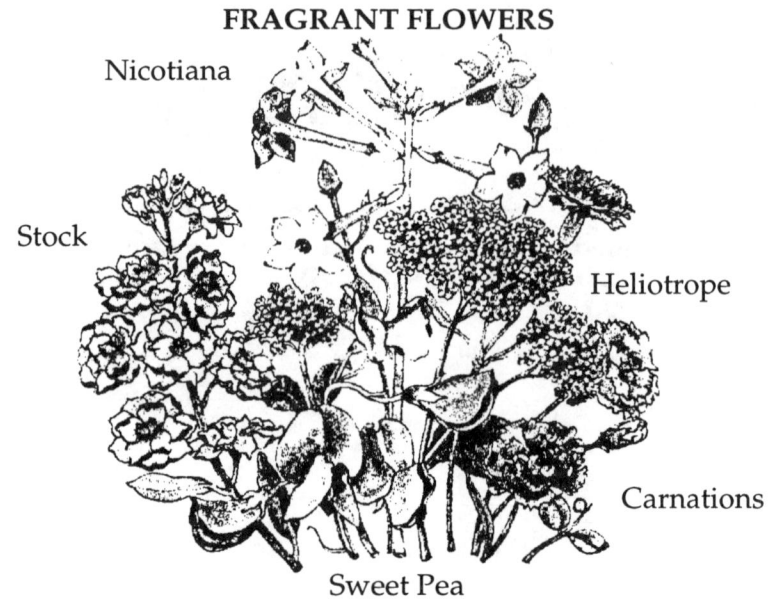

Nicotiana

Stock

Heliotrope

Carnations

Sweet Pea

OCTOBER

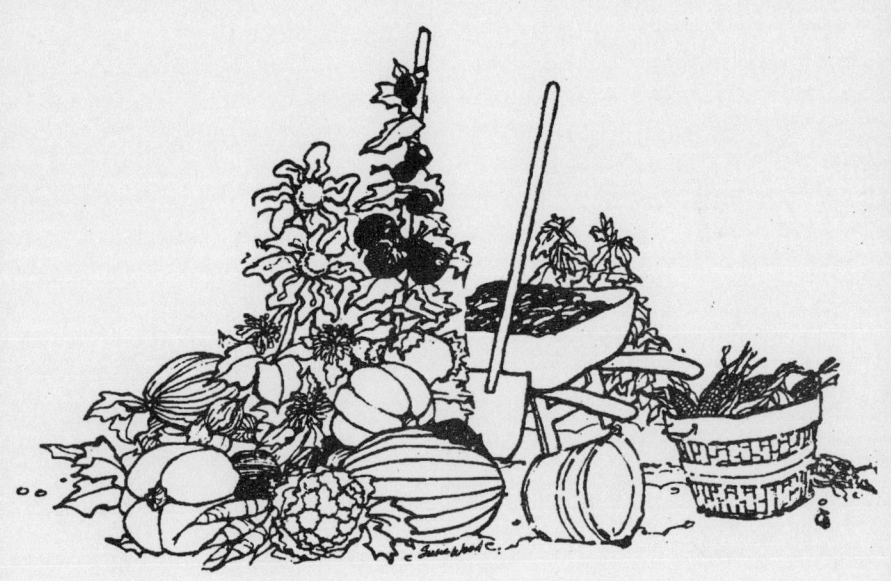

An abundance of vegetables gathered from the garden; as a harvest moon rises in the autumn sky.

OCTOBER

There's just a tinge of frost on the edges and a reminder of a garden wind-down. My garden does not freeze like a lot of gardens do. When the soil is in balance the life of the soil keeps the plants protected for a longer period of time. It's time to think of putting your garden to sleep. With a cover crop you protect the soil from wind and soil erosion and you build up nutrients for the coming year. I sprinkle wheat seed throughout my rows of vegetables, broccoli, cabbage and cauliflower. Just raking it in lightly to cover with soil gives it a start towards germination. As the wheat grows and the rest of the vegetables die and fade away, you always have a living, growing garden. This does many things the naked eye does not see. It prevents weed seeds from growing. It builds humus in the top six inches of soil. It protects the soil from erosion and provides nutrients that sometimes we can't measure. While this is quietly going on we are still harvesting a full thirty days yet. The vegetables we planted in July and August are now ready to harvest. What's nice about a fall garden is the crops linger because of the cool nights and do not go to seed. Only the true gardener knows the feeling of raising and serving vegetables and fruit grown by the sweat of the brow. Just some of the plants still producing in the garden are the radishes, lettuce, spinach and green onions served as a relish tray, surrounded by a meal of stir-fried vegetables of squash, broccoli, cauliflower, celery and eggplant. The tomato vines are loaded with fruit, ready to be canned into sauce or juice or stewed whole. There are so many ways the hearty tomato can be used. The famous B.L.T. sandwich is one. Tomatoes cooked together with zucchini squash, onion and okra with a touch of home grown basil as an herb flavor is a favorite of ours.

This is also clean-up time for small amounts of vegetables to be canned into soup. The bursted heads of cabbage, celery, onions and green beans...the list is endless of vegetables that taste good together. Freezing vegetable combinations is good for planning winter menus. Especially good is broccoli, cauliflower and carrots. They should be frozen in amounts according to family size. Not to be forgotten is the value of drying some foods for easier storage. Dehydrators are reasonable or a handyman can make his own. Today we have resources to read on ways of preserving food. When I first learned about the natural way of eating I often had to attend Natural Food Associate meetings to learn the correct way to preserve food. We persisted in growing food without chemicals and today this is being accepted, mainly because of the increase of degenerative diseases with no cure for many patients in advanced stages.

This month is also a time for fruit harvesting. Apples can be canned, frozen, juiced, made into sauces and sliced for pies and cobblers. When freezing, use the best size apples with the best texture. Canned apple slices are very handy when making pies, cakes and cobblers. Applesauce is so handy, ready from the jar. I don't peel these apples, I cut them in quarters and cook them in a small amount of water. Then I put them through a colander. The pink tone of the peeling makes an appetizing appeal. One must cold pack in a hot water bath for 15 minutes to seal the rubber of the Ball or Kerr lids. Ready made apple pies made with a whole wheat crust, and then frozen, makes a quick dessert for unexpected company.

Here's a recipe I use:

2 C. whole wheat flour   1 C. lard
2 C. unbleached flour

Mix until crumbly. Add 1 egg with enough water to make ½ cup, plus 1 tablespoon apple cider vinegar. Knead quite well before rolling out for a crust. Cut enough apples in slices for one pie. Mix in a dish with 2 tablespoons whole wheat flour and ½ cup honey. Spread in a pie shell, cover with a top crust, making holes with knife in pie dough. Brush with water or milk mixed with egg yolk to form a shine on top. I cut a 2" strips of cloth and wrap around the pie tin to prevent any juices from escaping. Bake 40 minutes at 325° or until apples are soft. This depends upon the type of apple you are using.

Another recipe:

2 C. apple juice   4 T. tapioca

Cook until clear, add 2 cups fresh shredded apples. Chill and pour into baked crust.

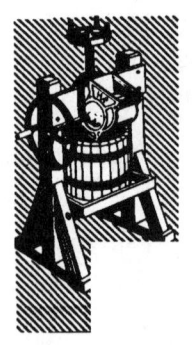

The most tedious job is making apple cider. They say the best is saved until last. This could be the case of the apple orchard. With a combination of apples all ripe now, that makes a better tasting cider. Extra help is always welcome for this chore. Drinking it fresh, of course, is the best. I can and freeze some to use later in the year. It seems like there is never room to freeze enough. After the jars are filled with juice I put them into a canner and bring the water to a boil just to seal the lids.

When we were introduced to the natural way of eating in 1959 there were seventeen acres on this farm that we purchased that were special to the previous owner. John O'Dell informed us of his childhood days spent in the area of the mouth of Fountain Spring. He said that this was the water that in 1855 turned the stones of the mill that ground the farmers' grain from 20 miles around. A school, a house and a barn were near the spring. All of those buildings were gone when we bought the farm, but John said we would always have water, walnuts, butternuts and apples. It is a quiet place with a bird sanctuary and a trout stream where trout stockers in 1992 reported it to be one of six trout streams in the state of Iowa that reproduces brown trout. It was special to John O'Dell and is special to me today. Our apples come from very old apple trees and some young trees there. We haven't planted any trees there in the thirty-four years we have been living here. The birds did a good job of planting these young trees in protective places near the spring. The natural habitat keeps the apples worm free. Our cattle keep the fallen apples cleaned up and provide their manure as fertilizer for the trees. All trees do not bear each year, but an abundance can always be depended upon. The bountiful nut harvest is an annual event, and of course the water is a daily pumping of four hundred gallons per minute. Yes...what a special place!

Another fruit grown in abundance in my garden is the everbearing red raspberry. In this fall month the berries are at their best. These plants were brought to my garden by Father Louis White. We started with one single row. Now the patch is eight feet wide. The reason I like everbearing plants is that you get two chances for harvesting. Sometimes mother nature doesn't work with you and a spring crop does not bear. So many times if a fall crop is good the following spring will also be good. Perishable fruit is better sold locally. Raising fruit without chemicals is an added advantage. A U-Pick-Your-Own patch could be advantageous but it would have to be a good sized patch of half an acre or more. I choose to pick my own patch because the canes can be broken off very easily when loaded with fruit. My satisfied customers always spread the word to other potential customers.

Concord grapes are also ripe now. I have never had a failure of grapes in my 34 years of gardening naturally. Of course you remember when we trimmed them in March to look for the bearing buds that were to be left on the vine. A needle nose pliers is a good tool that I have found to ease the job of cutting the stems of grapes. Grapes cannot be all picked at one time. The riper they are, the more true flavor you have. Most of my grapes are steamed and then hung in a cheesecloth sack to drip slowly. I put this concentrate into jars and seal them with

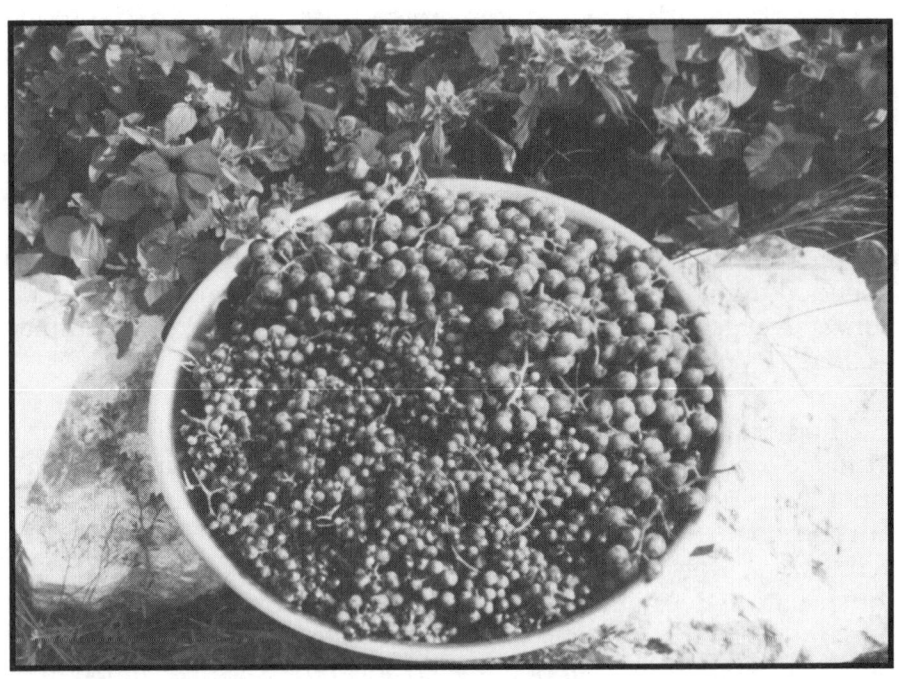
A combination of wild and tame grapes for concentrate.

Kerr or Ball lids, then bring to a boil in a hot water bath. When I use this in a drink I mix one half water and one half juice. We also like grape pie. For this I slip the pulp from the skins, boil the pulp till soft, then strain through a strainer. The seeds will separate from the pulp. Stir this pulp with the skins and package in containers for pies. When making the pies, heat this mixture for one pie with one half cup honey, 4 tablespoons arrowroot flour or one package of unflavored gelatin. As this cooks it will thicken. Pour into pie shell and cover with top crust.

This may be your last chance to cut your rhubarb one more time, that is, if you have continually removed the seed stalk. This makes a good juice to be mixed with apple or cherry juice. Once again the rhubarb is steamed, then put in a colander to drip. Pour juice concentrate in jars and put in a hot water bath for 10 minutes to seal the lid. From now on let the plant grow until frost. Juicing vegetables, using a combination with carrots, is a good way to use excess vegetables. Stir-frying can be another good source of using extra vegetables. Don't forget to add some type of herb in the juice and food for added taste and nutrition.

Nature's beauty is at its best this month. With the slight frost, the changing of the colors of the trees makes one be thankful for the different seasons. I consider myself lucky to be able to see the colors of the leaves changing every day from my kitchen window. Lucky also that those trees are in a county park which prevents them from being cut down. Generous local people donated the land to the county and made all this possible. Habitat and food for a lot of wildlife helps balance nature. Driving through this park on any one day you can see the native birds and animals. A pleasant camping area is available for vacation loving families. One of the highlights for Ralph and I was to drive through the park after Saturday night church services to visit with the campers and see if they got their allotment of fresh trout.

Back to the chore of this month which should be the dividing of the perennial flower beds. To enjoy a larger flower, and more of them, you should separate the root crowns of any perennials such as iris, lilies, peonies, lilacs, phlox, chrysanthemums, rhubarb and many more. Share your excess with a friend or neighbor or anyone who will plant them. Grape vines can be laid in the ground six inches deep. Leave the vine connected to the parent stock until new shoots appear the following spring. Grape vines need support to allow picking of the fruit.

Depending upon where you live, this is the time to plant spring blooming bulbs. In the northeast, Zone 4, where I live, this is the opportune time to plant tulips, daffodils and delphinium. A little mulch for protection helps nurse the plants through winter.

Drying vegetables is a growing method of preserving the last vegetable harvest. You can use the sun as a solar dryer, your oven on a low heat setting, or a dehydrator made especially for the job.

They sky will be clear with hardly a cloud in sight, the air will be sharp, the wind will be calm and the weather reports will be talking about frost. That's the moment you suddenly decide you cannot kiss your favorite geranium good-by, and it becomes hard to say farewell to the perennials that have bloomed all summer. We gather pots, cans, and crockery and stuff them two by two into any available nook and cranny indoors to reward us with blooms on our windowsill on cloudy winter days. Many hardy annuals do not winter over. In nature they need to blossom, set seed and then say farewell. Annual flowers like alyssum, marigolds, petunias, portulaca, grandflora and moss rose fall into this category. If mulch protection is placed on them now, they will reseed in spring. Most perennials need to have a sharp freeze to perform and blossom next year. Geraniums, impatiens, verbena, ivy and begonias are easy to dig up and repot for winter enjoyment. The size of the container depends on how much of the sprawling plant you want to bring indoors. Sharply pruning just above an "eye" where a new shoot is emerging will encourage new growth.

Some gardeners would rather snip off the old plant. To do this do not make your cuttings longer than four inches. The easiest way to iniate root cuttings is to place them in water in a dark colored glass or bottle, being sure to change the water frequently. As soon as roots appear, plant the cuttings one half to an inch deep in slightly moist peaty soil. Try to keep the soil damp, but not soggy wet until the roots have formed. I use two thirds garden soil and one third compost for potting my plants. The roots are dipped in a solution of fish emulsion of 3 tablespoons to one gallon of water. If watered with this solution after the plants are set out is a guarantee of survival. Early planting of the flowers you intend to keep indoors allows you to harden them off by leaving them outside until rooted. Then when watering and feeding your plants during winter I mix my own plant food:

1 tsp. baking powder	1 tsp. salt
1 tsp. salt peter	½ tsp. household ammonia

Mix in one gallon tepid water. Store in a glass jug. Water plants every 5 or 6 weeks with this solution.

Now that your perennials are house plants, they will require less water. A good rule of thumb is to let the soil dry out slightly between waterings. A constant soggy plant soon suffocates. Place in a south or east window where sunlight can feed them.

Soap making time for the entire year comes this month while you can still have windows open in the basement. Choose the dark of the moon to make perfect soap. My recipe is 6 pounds of melted tallow heated to lukewarm. Mix one can of lewis lye in two and a half pints of cold water in an enamel pan. Do not use plastic or aluminum. This will heat up so constant stirring is necessary. When both lye water and melted tallow are the same temperature pour one into the other and stir for five minutes. At this time I add dried rose petals from summer blooms for a rose scent to use in washing clothes. Stir again for five to ten minutes, until thick as pudding. Line a cardboard box with waxed paper and pour into the box. When partially set, cut in squares. The following day cut squares apart and let them dry out and then store.

The popcorn is now ready to pick. This must be laid out in shallow boxes to dry and cure. Storing indoors to dry free of dust and humidity is important. This process could be six to eight weeks.

A good way to use up your excess cabbage is by making sauerkraut. This is an old tradition and so easy to do. Shred the cabbage in a food processor, stuff it quite firmly into jars, add one tablespoon of salt to each quart, pour boiling water to fill the jar and poke a wooden spoon handle down the middle and sides to get as much water in as possible. Seal with a rubber and a zinc lid. To keep the sauerkraut snow white, store the jars in a canner wrapped in newspaper to absorb the moisture that works out from the lid. It should be ready for use in six weeks.

After the frost has killed the sweet potato vines it is time to dig them up. Storage is almost opposite the Pontaic or Cobbler. Sweet potatoes like a very warm place and should be wrapped in newspaper and placed in crates for air to reach them. They are high in Vitamins A and C.

Fall is a good time to plant trees. Plant a hardwood tree every year. Do you know the value of the tree other than its lumber? Here are some values:

Trees absorb carbon dioxide.
Trees provide shade. Trees that shade your house can cut your energy requirements for air conditioning by fifty percent.
Trees provide homes for wildlife.

Trees provide changing colors during the year.

Trees provide their weight in nitrogen each day.

Trees provide leaves for mulch which is a fertilizer that decomposes right where they fall.

Trees grow as you grow.

The story goes that a ten year old boy was asked what he knew about trees. His answer was "some trees have fruit and some trees have nuts, but some trees just stand there". Since the average American citizen uses seven trees a year it would be a gesture of love to replace them.

Just a few herbs grown in my garden, mostly for medicinal uses, are the famous comfrey plant, borage lemon balm, peppermint, sage, chives and nettle.

When we were first introduced to the natural way of living our skin was in a very bad state. There were sores in most creased places of our bodies. Little did we know that the combination of the toxic chemicals we were using was the cause of our problem. The doctors were treating the symptoms and not the cause of the severe itching and burning skin. Father Louis White taught me all that I know about gardening and the first remedy he suggested was a poultice of steeped comfrey leaves applied on a cheese cloth and then put on the body sores. We tied it with a bandage to keep it in place during the night. After doing this for three weeks the skin started to heal. We also steeped the leaves and added honey for a tea drink. Comfrey has been reported as a valuable medicinal herb in some of the old herbal books as far back as 200 A.D. But the first truly scientific report on comfrey was not published until 1936. The belief is that the leaves and roots of comfrey contain the priceless allantoin which is the healing agent. Allantoin has been used many years by the medical profession to stimulate healthy granulation of tissues. I know from experience that it is a healing plant. It healed all of our open sores, returning the skin to a healthy pink tone. This is the month to cut the comfrey leaves. Wash them gently and spread them out to dry on newspapers, away from dust. The leaves will take ten days to dry. Crumble them up and store them in a glass gallon jar. Use them in winter for tea or as a poultice when needed.

Borage was first planted in my garden to draw bees for pollination. Reading and studying about this plant I found that it had medicinal properties also. Steeping these leaves and applying them as a poultice in a cheese cloth on eyes that had welding burns or hay dust, or just tired eyes, is a great relief. It's also good for babies that develop cradle cap or sore eyes. Use a weaker solution for this and bathe gently. It can also increase the milk flow of nursing mothers when taken as a tea drink.

The mint family of peppermint, spearmint and lemon balm, combined as tea, are cool soothers on a hot day.

Chives, garlic, onion, parsley, sage and cilantra are all grown as flavorings in food, but they are also of medicinal value. A small root of each, potted in small clay pots, can give your winter menu a lift. All of these can be dried or frozen. A hint I have used is to chop the parsley and chives very fine, then add water and pour into an ice cube tray to freeze. This gives you just the right amount for making stews or soups. The cubes can be stored in a plastic bag or other container in the freezer.

I cut and dry stinging nettle to use as a rinse for my hair to keep the color. Steep a large handful of dried leaves in one quart of water. Use one cup per each hair washing. Keep the rest refrigerated for later use. It makes the hair soft and shiny.

This has been a busy month indeed, preparing for five months food storage until the next garden season.

Take time to enjoy the last blooms on the roses.

NOVEMBER

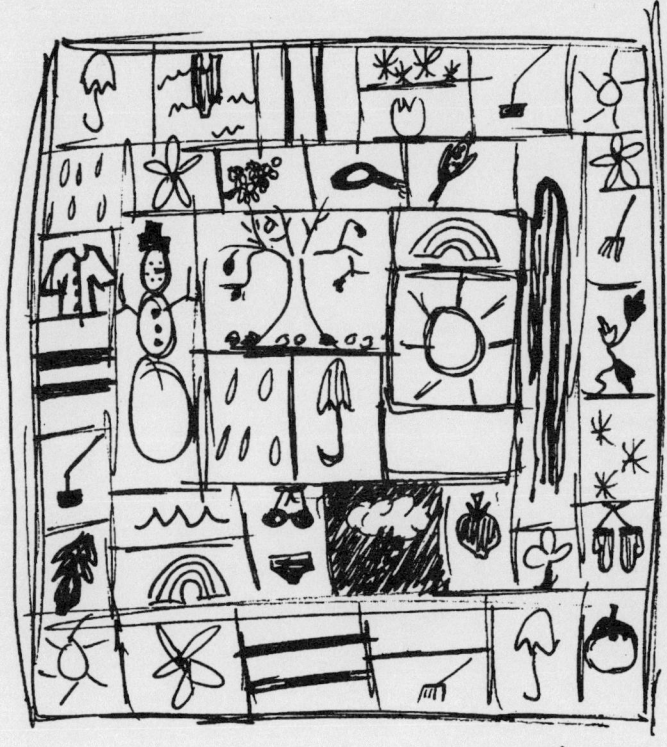

The rapid change from summer to fall,
makes us reflect and recall.
How seasons come and seasons go
to help make our gardens grow.

NOVEMBER

The garden produce is winding down but still the late fall crops have not frozen. I'm still cutting spinach, lettuce, broccoli and the root crops of turnips and radishes. There is plenty of work to be done to put the garden to rest. One big chore is to trim the everbearing red raspberry patch. I cut the live standing canes waist high, then all dead canes must be removed from the patch and burned. It is important to clean out the patch in this way. Dead canes could carry diseases and the berries could be crumbly the next year. The dead canes produced the spring crop. The soil does not get worked like the rest of the garden so we must provide hired hands of nature to aerate the soil. What can we do to get this soil in balance and aerated without tillage? We must rely on mother nature. Feed the soil and the soil will feed the plant. What I feel is an absolute must in my patch is Bio-Dynamic made compost spread through the entire patch. A one fourth inch layer is sufficient. I do this after the patch has been trimmed. I have poplar trees and huge soft maple shade trees that drop their leaves and nicely mulch my patch without any of my labor. This makes a secure bed for earthworms to have a comfortable home to apply their weight in nitrogen daily and the worms do the aerating of the soil when the temperature of the soil is fifty-five degrees. The earthworm is nature's own fertilizer factory. It not only eats dirt, but embraces all waste, both vegetable and animal. He swallows all that decaying matter voraciously. He digests by mixing rich secretions from his own digestive system and deposits this residue into the earth as castings. Laboratory analyses show these castings contain three times more magnesium, five times more nitrogen, seven times more phosphorus and eleven times more potash than ordinary soil. There is a law of demand which is give and take. You get out of your soil what you put into it. The earthworm labors valiantly to put back all the rich minerals, trace elements and organic materials that lie locked in decaying vegetable and animal matter. They are original tillers of the soil. Mother

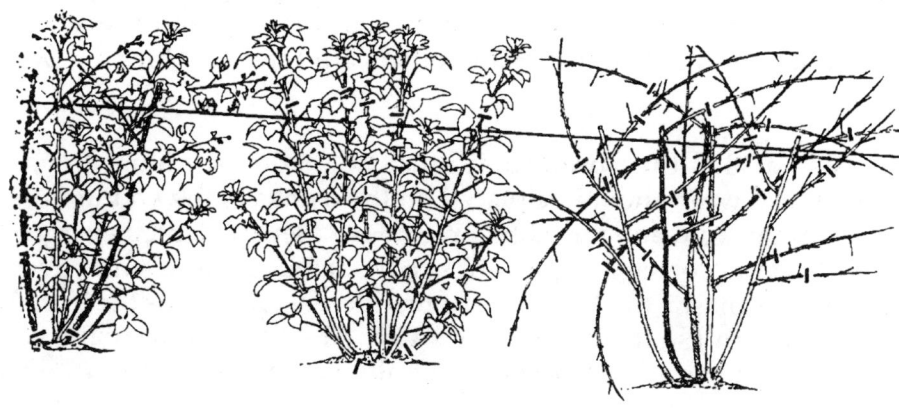

earth needs all these things to keep her metabolism at par. There is no waste in nature. When the tree has used what it needs for growth and production, the remainder of these minerals is carefully stockpiled in the leaves. Is it any wonder why we should compost our leaves instead of burning all our resources in smoke? Some other porous type of residue can now be applied to the raspberry patch. I use cornstalks that have been chopped. The leaves provide a blanket and the cornstalks allow air to go into and come out of the soil. A snow cover over these cornstalks provides moisture that is held and dispensed as weather and time permits. Some people use a trellis to hold up the canes. I never have and see no real use for them in my garden. A lot depends upon the type of berry you grow. The plants are still on the same location and weeds are not a problem, except for the grass creeping in from the lawn. I try to keep this heavily mulched with rotted straw or hay bales. Deciding which varieties to grow depends on your work schedule and your taste buds. I like the everbearing plants because of the continuing harvest from the same amount of space used to grow them.

Other chores left to put my garden to rest for the cold winter are cleaning the plants out and making a compost pile. The carrot tops, beet, turnip, lettuce and small residue plants are piled up. The tomato, potato, flowers and stalker residue is cut up with a mower. This helps to speed up decomposition. I layer it and put a shovel of dirt on every third or fourth layer. I use barnyard manure, cornstalk residue or any type of compostable material. I also mix a very small portion of B-D starter which is Dr. Pfeiffer's product and apply it between the layers. At this time of the year you will not get a heating action, but it will not lose the properties of the B-D starter. When the temperature gets to fifty five degrees the fifty five strains of micro-organisms will start to work. This is not the opportune time to make compost. This is a storage place for residue to be kept during the winter. One is surprised at the amount of vegetation still left in our gardens. All flowers are cut off or pulled out and placed on this compost pile. The phlox, peony, yarrow, comfrey and mums are all perennials and are cut off at ground level. The marigolds, zinnia, nasturtium and others are annuals which are pulled out.

Also at this time protection must be made for young trees. A commercial wrap should be placed on the trunks of the young trees to prevent sun scald and for rabbit protection. Newly planted evergreens need a wind protector to prevent needle damage to the small trees. I use a cutoff plastic tile 12 to 14" in circumference, as tall as the tree, dug into the ground so it will not blow away. Also at this time of the year I apply a ¼" layer of compost around all my fruit bearing trees which was made in July and August. This application is then covered with a mulch of either leaves or chopped corn stalks. What I am doing is protecting these live strains of micro-organisms against the extreme freezing-thawing cycle. These beneficial micro-organisms fight and destroy the eggs of the bad bugs which destroy our fruit. When the soil warms up to fifty-five degrees the eggs are starting to hatch in the soil, but the fifty-five strains of bacteria are also ready to work which prevent the destructive insects from maturing. I agree that maybe not all will be consumed but at this time we have mother nature's birds to help us. This layer of mulch will be eaten away when spring comes. We have this variety of insects chewing up the debris, and decomposition allows it to penetrate the soil.

Roses should be put to rest in November. The canes should be cut back to fourteen inches. Tie the canes together and mound the soil at least twelve inches over the bud union of each rose bush. Leave the top two inches exposed until the soil freezes. After the mound freezes, cover it with straw or evergreen boughs to keep the mound frozen. Cylinders of different material can be used. Wire mesh, bottomless bushel baskets, tar paper or burlap wrapping are all suggestions of materials to use. In my rose bed I put a mesh fence around the bed and fill this to cover the canes with leaves raked from the yard.

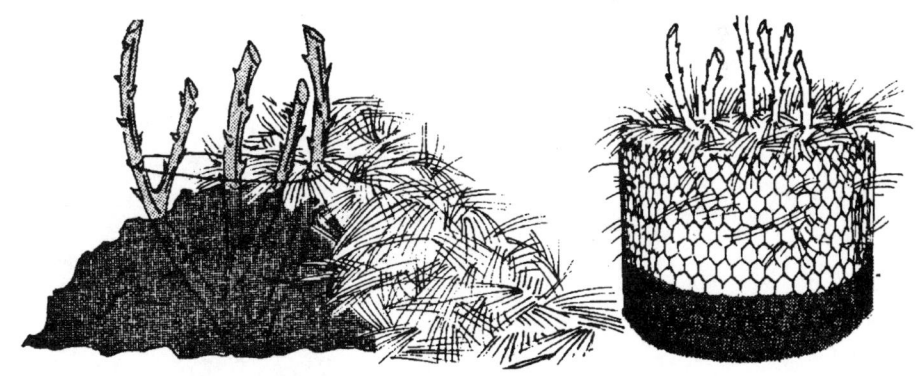

DECEMBER

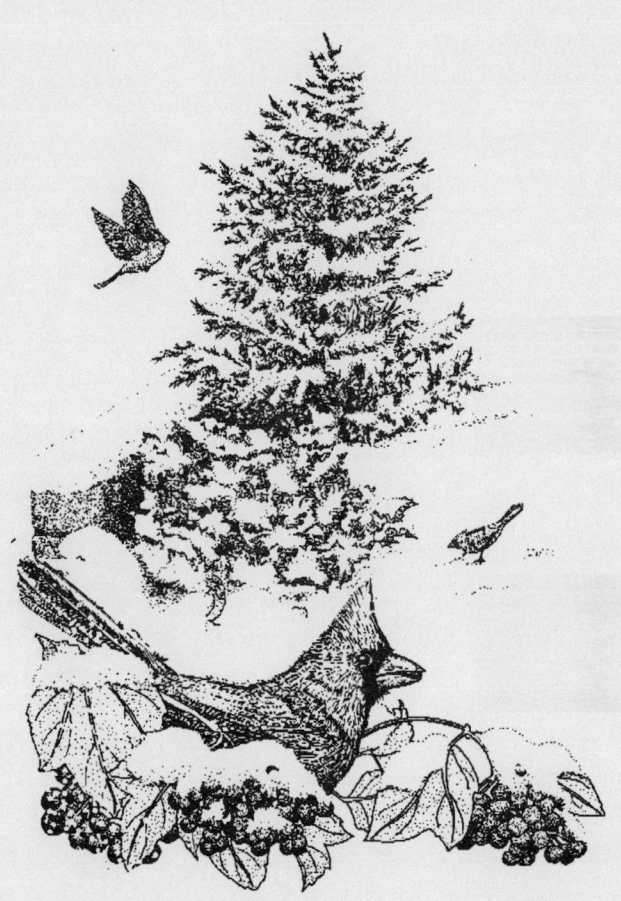

On the coldest wintery day;
Evergreen trees standing so tall
catching all of the snow that falls.
Providing a perfect nesting place
when a bird comes into space.

DECEMBER

Now we come to the month when the gardener is the farthest removed from the garden. No physical work can be done with the soil in the Midwest of the United States. This is the time for the soil to rest as nature planned from the very beginning of time. It is an interesting month, with the start of winter on December 22, and then the shortest day, with days giving us gradually less daylight hours. This month is time for ourselves to also take that rest from our daily lives, to look back on what we have accomplished in the past year. December is not a dull month by any means. We have clean, white snow to decorate our trees and landscape, sometimes sparkled with ice crystals that glitter in the sunlight. We have quiet times when we are snowed in by a foot of snow, when we can read a book or write a letter to a friend. We have the Christmas holiday to look forward to, friends visiting, families getting together and cards and messages coming in from around the world.

I was one of eight children, born in the Depression of the 1930s. We had no electricity, a wood stove for heat and our bedrooms had no heat at all. We milked our cows by hand and turned a crank separator by hand to separate the cream from the skim milk. The cream was stored in 10 gallon cans in a cooling tank with a constant flow of running water. The cream as taken to town 17 miles away to a creamery and made into butter. We soaked corn and oats in the skim milk in wooden barrels and fed it to our hogs. My parents did not own any property and always rented on a share basis. I can remember my father saying his rent was paid each night he went to bed. My mother talked about bartering eggs, cream, flour and sugar for rubber tires. My memories of Christmas as a little girl are very different from today's world. The Christmas tree was set up on December 24 by Santa. New ornaments were added each year. Each of the eight children had their place at the table and at each place was a Christmas gift from Santa. They consisted of school writing paper, pencils, new barrettes for your hair, your own bag of candy or an orange for Christmas breakfast. Most of the toys were made of tin or wood. The dolls had stuffed straw bodies with a breakable china head. After looking at the gifts we received we all had our chores to do.

The children stayed home to help their parents with the work until they started their life with their partner. Even through the Depression we always had enough food to eat. Maybe not a lot of choices, but food to grow and sustain us. School was seventeen miles from our farm. My father drove us each day to school, then picked us up at 3:30 p.m. The country school had closed and at that time no one heard of a school bus to pick up the children. We had to walk one mile each day to pick up our daily mail, then one mile back home. We could survive and live on much less than we have today. Ours was a happy family. I cannot remember being depressed or stressed out as it is referred to today. Those were trying times for our parents and today the problems are still with us, but in a different way and at a greater level.

Many of the ideas from my growing up and working with my mother in her garden are still being practiced in my garden today. December is the time to appreciate the food we toiled with the past year. A trip to my food cellar provides any meal I want to serve. The frozen food I prepared throughout the year is like going to a grocery store and choosing the menu for the day. The potatoes, squash, onions and garlic which have been grown, dug and stored are staple foods we eat each day. The cabbage, Chinese cabbage, turnips and carrots are added dishes to our menu. The cabbage was wrapped in cellophane and stored in a refrigerator in the basement. Turnips and carrots are stored in tubs and then covered with soil to seal them over. This part of our basement has no heat, but the walls are insulated. The keeping quality is very good up until May first. I believe the way the food is grown has a lot of bearing on how well it keeps. As I have said so often, all life comes from the soil. To sustain life we must grow food with life so we can be bodily nourished with food with life in it. A real treat is the strawberries, rhubarb and raspberries in December. They have a fresh flavor when served just as they are thawed. Additional ways to enjoy them are over whole wheat short cake, as a syrup over whole wheat pancakes or whipped in a blender for a breakfast drink.

With the variety of frozen and canned vegetables no meal should be hard to plan. Each year I try some new vegetable and usually it becomes a favorite by year's end. I remember when the Sugar Snap pea was introduced to gardeners some fifteen years ago. Now it is a staple vegetable in my garden. Used in stir-fry vegetables or eaten fresh in lettuce salads or steamed as a hot vegetable is common in most family meals. What a lot of home gardeners have forgotten is the value of our home raised food. We put our energy into planting, growing, harvesting and preserving the food and then again handling the food in preparing our meals. We also know how it was carefully raised without toxic chemicals. We worked with the plants daily, watching the growth patterns and we nurtured them with tender loving care as we would with a growing child.

When the gardener has extra vegetables or fruits they are usually shared with friends, bartered for something you cannot raise. There is a growing demand for home raised fruits and vegetables grown without chemicals. Marketing still needs to be worked on. Organizations are cropping up all over the United States and the world for a better marketing system. Certification programs are increasing, some with better results than others. A tighter restriction must be made on the companies that manufacture carcinogenic substances. If a product is restricted and toxic, it must not be used, even if there are schools that certify those who attend and pass the requirements for applying the products to their croplands. We must remember that what we put into the soil creates a chain reaction and as humans we are the last in the chain to consume the food and be harmed. I recall many of my conversations with the late Fr. Louis P. White and his standing ovation comment was "Take care of nature and nature will take are of you." Fr. White was so far advanced in his knowledge that most people could not believe him. Today, 35 years later, the very things he talked about are coming true; like the bottled water he preached to his parishioners we would be buying over the counter because what was in our wells would be unfit to drink. He also stated many times that the food we would buy would not be safe to eat because of the overuse and misuse of toxic, restricted chemicals. Just think back to the cases of the Alar apple spray, the sulfate in our salad bars and the nitrates in our water. During his prime time in life there was not much support from universities, the Extension, government programs, churches or the people themselves. Today changes are being accepted. But too much damage has been done already. It will now take each of us to combine our efforts to make changes. I can remember Fr. White pleading with me to change my way of cooking and then my way of gardening and then myself educating by reading books and attending meetings to lead us toward farming and gardening without chemicals. Fr. White did not criticize us too much on using chemicals but came down hard on us to open our minds and listen to what others were already doing. We had many problems with our health and the health of our then seven children. As we attended these meetings and talked with other families who had similar problems, we began to have more courage to change our way of life.

Through this entire book I want to encourage you readers to take advantage of the opportunities out there. The road has been paved for the beginner to change his ways to growing food the natural way. I think of my life as a crusader to prove health can be restored to soil and in turn make the world healthier in which to live.

During my travels to Canada, Latvia and Siberia I taught the private farmers and gardeners the benefits of composting. Composting is death and decay of residue which is returned to earth to provide humus for rebirth of another crop. The residue also needs some quiet time to rebuild strength to complete its job in the soil. It is not a new practice at all, but an old art that needs to be revived. We lived in a time of a waste and throw-away society. Well, not so anymore. anyone can begin to recycle compostable waste. Just think about it for a moment. The deep roots of a 20 year old tree must bring up many minerals to form the leaves on this tree. The leaf will live the entire year, drop to the ground in fall and die and decay naturally to fertilize that same tree for the following year. Every year you see decay and rebirth. Take a lesson from nature and apply that to growth in plant life. Of course we must help along. Our fields are not in the forest so we must watch for tell-tale signs. Learn the deficiency signs from your plants. I like to see a deep dark green color in the night shade plants like tomatoes and potatoes. Yellowish leaves indicates stress because of a deficiency.

During this month of December we should take time to read good books, educating ourselves on specific subjects. Another uplifting chore in December is bird feeding. Some trees can be grown for natural feeding, such as the Mountain Ash and the Juniper tree. Most of us know that some of the best insecticides we can get are our feathered friends, the birds. Try to work with the birds that inhabit your yard during the year and then reach out for other birds. Birds make a winter garden brighter and livelier. Three essential items for their existence are food, water and shelter. Because shelter is so important we should plant vines, shrubs and trees for them. Without this protection the birds will choose the wild. Berry shrubs and fruiting trees are a prime source of food for our feathered friends. The Red Cedar gives a continuing supply of berries and the Hawthorn keeps its fruit well into spring. Robins

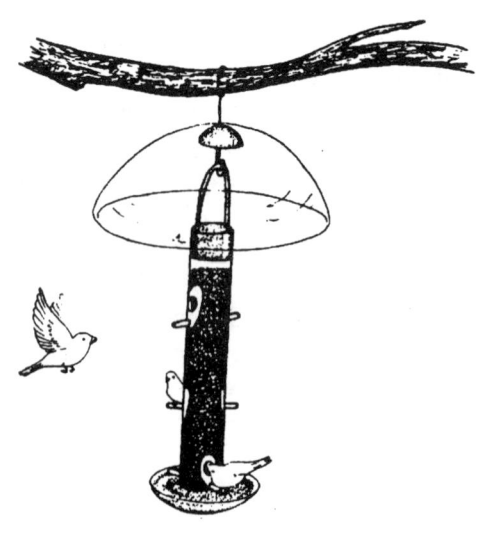

feast on holly berries when it is too early to find worms. Birds favor Dog Woodberries in all seasons. Cedar Waxwings like the blue black fruit of the Virginia Creeper and flowering crabs. Most birds devour insects, but eat berries in all seasons. When these cannot be provided, be kind to your silent workers and keep well filled feeders in your yard where you can see and enjoy them. The Purple Finch, along with the

Goldfinch are avid feeders of Niger seed. A mixture of Cedar Waxwings, Cardinals, Blue Jays, Finches and Snowbirds in my back yard is reason enough to plant habitat that draws and keeps the birds coming.

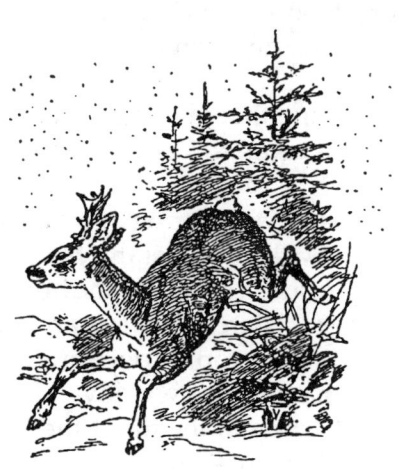

Deer hunting is another winter sport in our Delaware County. With increasing damage caused by deer to young trees, large round bales and agricultural crops such as corn, deer hunting is almost a necessity. The sport is enjoyed by my sons who are fortunate to get their limit each year. Along with hunting comes the processing of the carcasses. The group designates a place to cut, grind and package the deer. Our basement is the usual meeting place where we have the cutting and grinding machines. Deer that is hunted on your own property is usually corn fed from standing corn or self fed from the alfalfa round bales. The meat is processed as each family desires. Our favorites are deer hamburger, canned deer meat and deer steaks. It is a lean meat and very tender.

Other garden related chores are the trimming and watering of my herbs and house plants. The herbs are dug up in the fall with only a small portion of a root to grow fresh herbs during the winter. Sage is used in cooking. Potted parsley gives a nice garnish to your winter meals.

Plant food for potted flowers (keep it indoors) is made as you use it. Mix into one gallon of water:

1 tsp. baking powder   ½ tsp. household ammonia
1 tsp. Epsom salt   1 oz. compost
1 tsp. salt peter

Stir together and use to water every six weeks.

My flowers were also dug up and potted in garden soil to bloom and to take slips from to be rooted for the following year. Geraniums bloom for me all winter long. The waxy leaves of Begonias which have been brought in from my rock garden give a variety of color and texture. My best results in taking slips for the next year are when they are taken when there is a full moon. A green colored glass or bottle produces roots quicker than a clear bottle. A sweet potato vine grown all winter provides the slips we need to set out in the spring, plus the lovely vine. Plants, sets or seeds saved from your own garden is a savings. But more than the savings, I like the idea of getting a particular strain of gene from my own seeds.

We find that plants get balanced to the soil and resist disease. Caution must be taken to keep the seed clean for planting next season.

An early gathering of walnuts that are now dried is another so called chore. With extra baking for the holidays, walnuts are a tasty addition to any recipe, especially the home made fudge and other candies, cookies and pies. There is always an ample supply of walnuts to be harvested. My bumper crop of popcorn also needs to be hand peeled; a pleasant job on a quiet, snowy day. The handpeeling allows you to discard the small kernels at the tip of the ear. Pouring the corn from one container to another on a windy day gets rid of the chaff. Usually if the corn shells good it is dry enough for storage. I store mine in gallon glass jars. This makes a nice Christmas gift when put in unique glass containers.

Decorating the house for Christmas is done with live evergreen branches. Pruning these branches keeps shaping the tree and also gives an evergreen scent in our home. Discard these branches by laying them on the strawberry bed. This holds the moisture as the snow melts and gives the birds a playground and wind protection.

As the twelve months of a busy year are over we look back to what we can change to be a better gardener. Our main interest must always be, to be a good steward of the soil. I have dedicated my last 40 years learning ways to work with nature. I hope this book has given the reader some helpful insights on what can be done. Set a goal! Learn from your mistakes. Then spread the word so others too may share your knowledge.

COMPANION PLANTS

Combinations of vegetables, herbs, flowers and weeds that are mutually beneficial, according to current reports of organic gardeners and companion planting traditions.

PLANTS	COMPANIONS AND EFFECTS
Asparagus	Tomatoes, parsley, basil
Basil	Tomatoes (improves growth and flavor); said to dislike rue; repels flies and mosquitoes.
Beans	Potatoes, carrots, cucumbers, cauliflower, cabbage, summer savory, most other vegetables and herbs; around houseplants when set outside.
Beans (bush)	Sunflowers (beans like partial shade, sunflowers attract birds and bees), cucumbers (combination of heavy and light feeders), potatoes, corn, celery, summer savory.
Beets	Onions, kohlrabi.
Borage	Tomatoes (attracts bees, deters tomato worm, improves growth and flavor), squash, strawberries.
Cabbage Family	Potatoes, celery, dill, chamomile, sage, thyme, mint, pennyroyal, rosemary, lavender, beets, onions. Aromatic plants deter cabbage worms.
Carrots	Peas, lettuce, chives, onions, leeks rosemary, sage, tomatoes.
Catnip	Plant in borders; protects against flea beetles.

Celery	Leeks, tomatoes, bush beans, cauliflower, cabbage.
Chamomile	Cabbage, onions.
Chervil	Radishes (improves growth and flavor).
Chives	Carrots, plant around base of fruit trees to discourage insects from climbing trunk.
Corn	Potatoes, peas, beans, cucumbers, pumpkin, squash.
Cucumbers	Beans, corn, peas, radishes, sunflowers.
Dill	Cabbage (improves growth and health), carrots.
Eggplant	Beans.
Fennel	Most plants are supposed to dislike it.
Flax	Carrots, potatoes.
Garlic	Roses and raspberries (deter Japanese beetle); with herbs to enhance their production of essential oils; plant liberally throughout garden to deter pests.
Horseradish	Potatoes (deter potato beetle); around plum trees to discourage curculois)
Lamb's-quarters	Nutritious edible weed; allow to grow in modest amounts in the corn.
Leek	Onions, celery, carrots.

Lettuce	Carrots and radishes (lettuce, carrots and radishes make a strong companion team), strawberries, cucumbers.
Marigolds	The workhouse of pest deterrents. Keeps soil free of nematodes; discourages many insects. Plant freely throughout garden.
Marjoram	Here and there in garden.
Mint	Cabbage family; tomatoes; deters cabbage moth.
Mole plant	Deters moles and mice if planted here and there throughout the garden.
Nasturtium	Tomatoes, radishes, cabbage, cucumbers; plant under fruit trees. Deters aphids and pests of cucurbits.
Onion	Beets, strawberries, tomato, lettuce (protects against slugs), beans (protects against ants), summer savory.
Parsley	Tomato, asparagus.
Peas	Squash (when squash follows peas up trellis), plus grows well with almost any vegetable; adds nitrogen to the soil.
Petunia	Protects beans; benedicial throughout garden.
Pigweed	Brings nutrients to topsoil; benedicial growing with potatoes, onions and corn; keep well thinned.

Potato	Horseradish, beans, corn, cabbage, marigold, limas, eggplant (as trap crop for potato beetle).
Pot marigold	Helps tomato, but plant throughout garden as deterrent to asparagus beetle, tomato worm and many other garden pests.
Pumpkin	Corn.
Radish	Peas, nasturtium, lettuce, cucumbers; a general aid in repelling insects.
Rosemary	Carrots, beans, cabbage, sage; deters cabbage moth, bean beetles and carrot fly.
Rue	Roses and raspberries; deters Japanese beetle. Keep it away from basil.
Sage	Rosemary, carrots, cabbage, peas, beans; deters some insects.
Southernwood	Cabbage; plant here and there in garden.
Soybeans	Grows with anything; helps everything.
Spinach	Strawberries.
Squash	Nasturtium, corn.
Strawberries	Bush beans, spinach, borage, lettuce (as a border).
Summer Savory	Beans, onions. Deters bean beetles.
Sunflower	Cucumbers.

Tansy	Plant under fruit trees; deters pests of roses and raspberries; deters flying insects; also Japanese beetles, striped cucumber beetles, squash bugs; deters ants.
Tarragon	Good throughout garden.
Thyme	Here and there in garden; deters cabbage worm.
Tomato	Chives, onion, parsley, asparagus, marigold, nasturtium, carrot, limas.
Turnip	Peas.
Valerian	Good anywhere in garden.
Wormwood	As a border, keeps animals from the garden.
Yarrow	Plant along borders, near paths, near aromatic herbs; enhances essential oil.

SYSTEMS OF MINERAL ELEMENT DEFICIENCY IN PLANTS

Deficient element	Plant as a Whole	Leaves	Stems	Roots	Fruit
NITROGEN	Stunted in growth,	Relatively small thin, yellowish green or light lemon color. Red or purple veins.	Slender, woody light to yellow green.	Stunted, but usually proportionately less so than the the tops.	Fruit chlorotic; develope slowly. Small when mature, often brilliant red (apples). Seeds light in weight.
PHOSPHORUS	Slow growing, often drawfed at maturity.	Dark green color red leaf veins enhanced. Irregularly distributed brown patches common.	Slender, relatively woody.	Stunted, often proportionately less so than tops.	Fruits slow ripening; relatively small. Seeds late maturing and relatively light in weight.
POTASSIUM	Plants at first stunted, later dry up to a brownish color.	Dull green, sometimes yellow, edges and tips often scorched. Bronze-color spots develop. Older leaves affected first.	Usually slender, often with brown streaks.	Usually slender.	Seeds often fail mature. When they do, relatively, small in size.
SULFUR		Yellowish chlorosis showing first along veins in some species.	Often relatively slender, sometimes elongate.		

For additional information or for purchasing a book contact:

Engelken Garden Supply

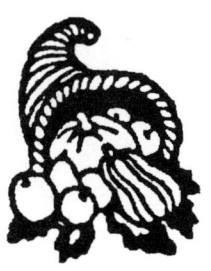

Rita Engelken
2478 135th Street
Greeley, Iowa 52050-8542
(319) 925-2962